Pancreatitis Diet
COOKBOOK

COMPREHENSIVE 21-DAY PANCREATITIS MANAGEMENT PLAN | CONTROL CHRONIC PAIN, REDUCE INFLAMMATION, AND SAVOR HEALTHY TASTY RECIPES WITH 200+ ESSENTIAL MEALS

RUBY A. STROTHERS

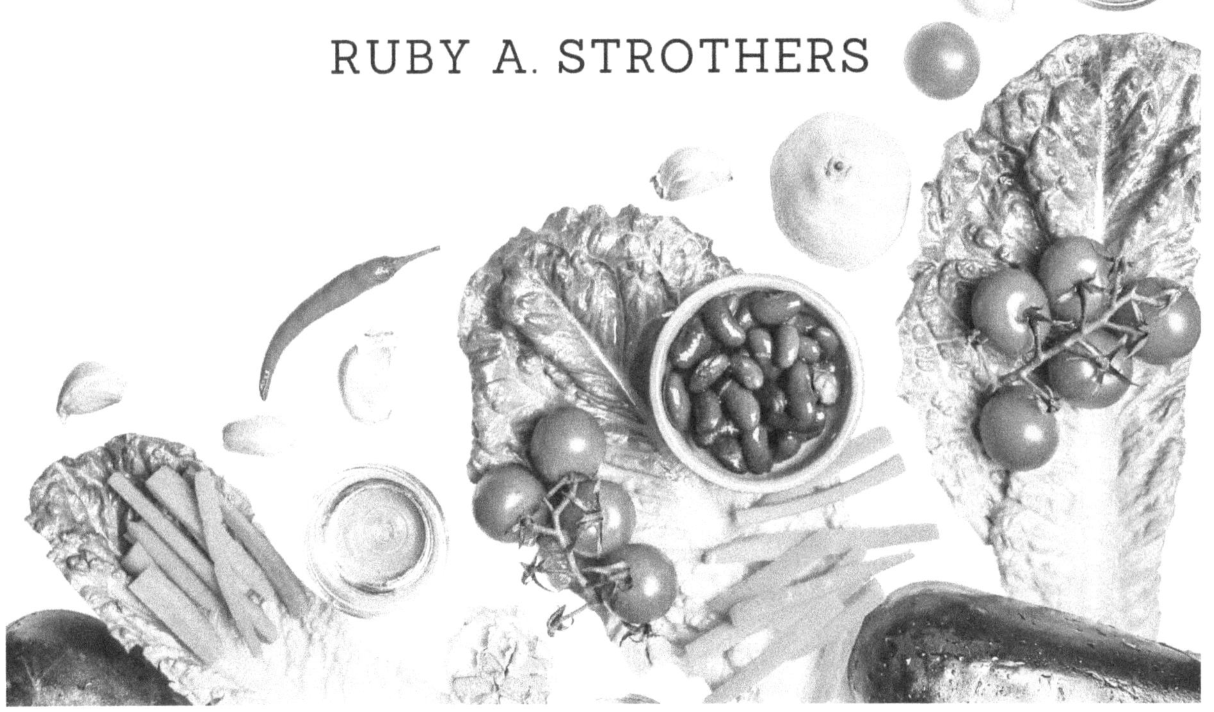

Your Opinion Matters!

Copyright © Ruby A. Strothers Publication

Kindly share your review if you enjoy this book and help us to create better products for you.

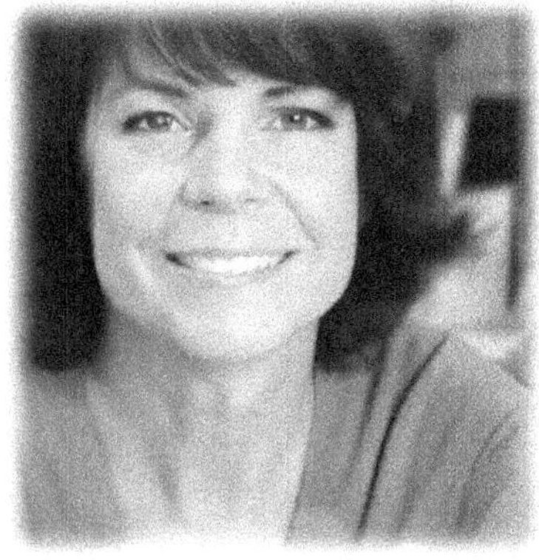

Ruby A. Strothers is a nutritionist, weight loss expert, and researcher who is passionate about helping people live a sustainable, healthy life through her resourceful cookbook and diet plan. She was born and raised in a small town in the United States and grew up with a keen interest in food and cooking.

After completing her education in nutrition and dietetics, Ruby A. Strothers started her career as a researcher, focusing on the relationship between food and weight loss. She spent several years conducting research studies and analyzing data to identify the most effective ways to help people lose weight and maintain a healthy lifestyle.

As a nutritionist and weight loss expert, Ruby A. Strothers has helped thousands of people lose weight and improve their overall health. She is known for her practical, science-based approach to weight loss, which emphasizes the importance of a balanced diet and regular exercise. She also believes in the power of mindfulness and stress reduction techniques, which can help people overcome emotional eating and other unhealthy habits.

In addition to her work as a nutritionist and researcher, Ruby A. Strothers is also a passionate cook and has written several cookbooks that are focused on healthy, sustainable eating. Her cookbooks are filled with delicious and easy-to-follow recipes that are designed to help people lose weight without sacrificing flavor or satisfaction.

Ruby A. Strothers is committed to helping people live a healthier, happier life, and she continues to be a leading voice in the field of nutrition and weight loss. Whether through her research, her cookbooks, or her counselling services, she is dedicated to helping people achieve their weight loss goals and maintain a healthy lifestyle for years to come.

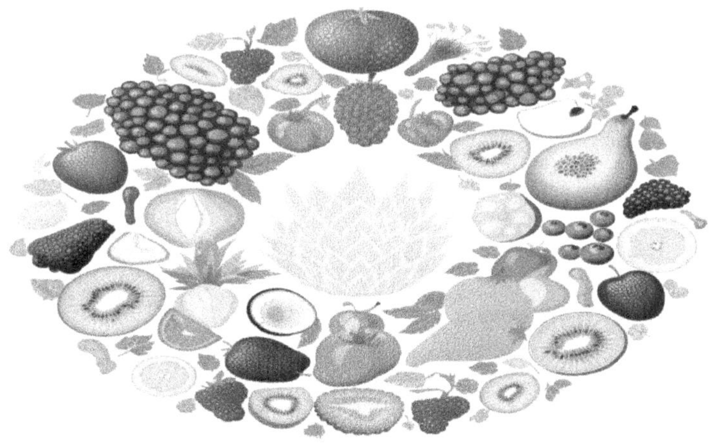

Contents

Welcome to the "Pancreatitis Diet Cookbook"! This comprehensive guide is designed to provide you with essential knowledge and delicious recipes tailored specifically for individuals managing pancreatitis.

Pancreatitis is a condition defined by inflammation of the pancreas, a vital organ responsible for generating enzymes to aid in digestion and supress blood sugar. When the pancreas evolves into inflamed, it can lead to severe abdominal pain, digestive issues, and potentially serious complications.

Managing pancreatitis often involves making significant dietary adjustments to alleviate symptoms and support the healing process. This cookbook aims to empower you with a wealth of culinary options that are not only nutritious but also gentle on the pancreas.

Within these pages, you'll find a collection of carefully crafted recipes curated by health and nutrition experts. These recipes prioritize ingredients that are easy on the pancreas, helping to reduce inflammation and provide necessary nutrients while ensuring delicious flavors and satisfying meals.

The journey to managing pancreatitis through diet can be daunting, but this cookbook serves as your reliable companion, offering:

- **Understanding Pancreatitis:** Insights into what pancreatitis is, its causes, symptoms, and the importance of diet in managing the condition.
- **Nutrition Guidance:** Detailed information on nutrients that are beneficial for pancreatic health and tips on selecting foods that support a pancreatitis-friendly diet.
- **Recipe Diversity:** A wide array of recipes ranging from comforting soups and light salads to hearty mains and delightful desserts, all carefully crafted to align with a pancreatitis-friendly diet.
- **Practical Tips:** Helpful suggestions on meal planning, portion control, ingredient substitutions, and strategies to make cooking enjoyable and stress-free.
- **Empowerment:** Guidance on how to adapt these recipes to fit personal preferences and dietary needs while adhering to the principles of a pancreatitis-friendly diet.

Whether you are newly diagnosed with pancreatitis or seeking ways to manage your symptoms effectively, this cookbook is your go-to resource for nourishing and flavorful meals. Each recipe is designed with your health and taste buds in mind, ensuring that you can savor meals without compromising on nutrition or exacerbating pancreatic issues.

Remember, this cookbook is a tool to support your journey towards better health, but it's essential to consult with your a registered dietitian for personalized guidance tailored to your specific health needs.

Get ready to commence on a culinary adventure that prioritizes your well-being without sacrificing the joy of good food. Let's cook our way to a healthier, happier you with the "Pancreatitis Diet Cookbook"!

Pancreatitis is a bodily state characterized by inflammation of the pancreas, an organ form behind the stomach. The pancreas performs a pivotal role in digestion by fabricating enzymes that help break down food and hormones like insulin to generate blood sugar levels.

There are two main kinds of pancreatitis: acute pancreatitis and chronic pancreatitis.

Acute Pancreatitis:

Acute pancreatitis is a instant inflammation of the pancreas that can compass from mild discomfort to severe, life-threatening illness.

It occurs when digestive enzymes become activated within the pancreas, causing damage to the pancreatic tissue. Gallstones and excessive alcohol consumption are common causes.

Symptoms of acute pancreatitis comprise severe abdominal ache that may radiate to the back, nausea, vomiting, and fever. Seek rapid medical assistance if these symptoms occur.

Chronic Pancreatitis:

Chronic pancreatitis refers a long-term inflammation of the pancreas that does not resolve and often leads to permanent damage.

Repeated episodes of acute pancreatitis, long-term alcohol abuse, certain genetic factors, and conditions like cystic fibrosis can contribute to chronic pancreatitis.

Symptoms include persistent abdominal pain, weight loss, oily or greasy stools (steatorrhea), and diabetes due to impaired insulin production.

Both types of pancreatitis can have severe consequences and require proper medical management. Treatment often involves hospitalization, pain management, intravenous fluids, and nutritional support. In some cases, surgery may be necessary to remove blockages or damaged tissue.

A pancreatitis diet is crucial in managing the condition and minimizing symptoms. It typically involves:

- Limiting alcohol consumption or abstaining entirely.
- Eating smaller, more periodic meals to ease the workload on the pancreas.
- Avoiding high-fat foods that can trigger attacks and exacerbate symptoms.
- Emphasizing a diet rich in fruits, vegetables, lean proteins, and whole grains.
- Working nearly with a healthcare professional or registered dietitian to tailor a diet plan based on individual needs.

The Pancreas Composition and its vital bodily role

The pancreas is a vital organ in our body with dual functions: exocrine and endocrine. Structurally, it's made up of glandular tissue and is situated behind the stomach, close to the small intestine. Its unique composition and location enable it to carry out crucial roles essential for proper digestion and blood sugar regulation.

Exocrine Function

The majority of the pancreas is dedicated to its exocrine function, producing enzymes that aid in digestion. These digestive enzymes, including amylase, lipase, and proteases, are released into the small intestine. They break down carbohydrates, fats, and proteins from the food we eat, facilitating their absorption and utilization by the body.

Endocrine Function

Within the pancreas are clusters of cells refers islets of Langerhans. These cells play a pivotal role in the organ's endocrine function by producing hormones. The two main hormones secreted by these islets are insulin and glucagon. They help regulate blood sugar levels by balancing the amount of glucose present in the bloodstream. Insulin lessens blood sugar levels by facilitating the intake of glucose into cells for energy, while glucagon raises blood sugar levels by signaling the release of stored glucose into the bloodstream when needed.

The pancreas is integral to maintaining the body's overall health by ensuring proper digestion and regulating blood sugar levels. Any dysfunction or damage to the pancreas, such as in the case of pancreatitis, can significantly impact these essential functions, leading to digestive issues and disturbances in blood sugar control.

Unveiling causes and signs of pancreatitis

Pancreatitis is a condition described by inflammation in the pancreas, a vital organ responsible for generating enzymes essential for digestion and hormones such as insulin for regulating blood sugar levels. Understanding the root causes and recognizing symptoms is crucial for managing this condition effectively.

Root Causes of Pancreatitis

- **Gallstones:** One of the most common causes, gallstones can block the pancreatic duct, triggering inflammation.
- **Alcohol Consumption:** Chronic and excessive alcohol intake can lead to pancreatitis by causing damage to pancreatic cells.
- **Smoking:** Cigarette smoking elevates the risk of developing pancreatitis.
- **Genetics:** Inherited disorders like cystic fibrosis and hereditary pancreatitis can elevate the risk.
- **High Triglyceride Levels:** Elevated levels of triglycerides in the blood can also lead to pancreatitis.
- **Certain Medications:** Some medications, especially certain antibiotics, can trigger pancreatitis in some individuals.
- **Trauma or Injury:** Physical trauma to the abdomen can cause inflammation in the pancreas.

Symptoms of Pancreatitis

* **Abdominal Pain:** Severe, dull pain in the upper abdomen or back, often worsened after eating or drinking.
* **Nausea and Vomiting:** Feeling poorly to the stomach and recurrent vomiting are common symptoms.
* **Fever and Rapid Pulse:** Inflammation may cause a fever and an increased heart rate.
* **Tender Abdomen:** The abdomen might feel tender or swollen to the touch.
* **Loss of Appetite:** A reduced inclination to eat due to discomfort or pain.
* **Jaundice:** Yellowish skin and eyes may occur if the bile duct becomes blocked due to inflammation.
* **Changes in Bowel Movements:** Oily, foul-smelling stools might indicate issues with fat digestion.

Recognizing these symptoms early and seeking medical attention is vital. Acute pancreatitis can progress rapidly and become life-threatening if not promptly treated. Long-term complications may arise, leading to chronic pancreatitis, which requires ongoing management and dietary adjustments.

Exploring diverse diseases linked to the pancreas

The pancreas, an organ crucial for digestion and hormone regulation, can be affected by various health conditions other than pancreatitis. Here are some other pancreas-related diseases:

Pancreatic Cancer

This is a serious condition where abnormal cells grow uncontrollably in the pancreas. It's often diagnosed at later stages, making treatment challenging. Risk factors include smoking, obesity, family history, and certain genetic conditions.

Pancreatic Insufficiency

This occurs when the pancreas doesn't produce enough digestive enzymes, leading to difficulties in digesting food. Conditions like cystic fibrosis, chronic pancreatitis, or pancreatic cancer can cause this insufficiency.

Diabetes

The pancreas plays a pivotal role in regulating blood sugar by producing insulin. In diabetes, the pancreas either doesn't generate enough insulin (Type 1) or the body grows resistant to insulin's effects (Type 2), leading to elevated blood sugar levels.

Acute Pancreatitis

While you're focusing on a pancreatitis diet cookbook, it's worth mentioning that acute pancreatitis is a unexpected inflammation of the pancreas, often caused by gallstones or excessive alcohol consumption. It requires immediate medical attention and typically resolves with treatment.

Chronic Pancreatitis

This is a indelible inflammation of the pancreas, often associated with prolonged alcohol use, certain genetic conditions, or blockages in the pancreatic duct. It leads to persistent pain, digestive issues, and can affect the pancreas' ability to function properly.

Pancreatic Pseudocyst

Sometimes, after an episode of pancreatitis, a fluid-filled sac (pseudocyst) can develop near the pancreas. While some resolve on their own, others might need drainage or medical intervention.

Pancreatic Fistula

This occurs when an abnormal connection forms between the pancreas and other organs or the skin, leading to the leakage of pancreatic fluids. It can happen after surgeries or as a complication of severe pancreatitis.

Coping strategies for acute pancreatitis

Coping with acute pancreatitis involves a multifaceted approach that requires immediate medical attention, dietary changes, lifestyle modifications, and careful management. Acute pancreatitis is a condition characterized by the sudden inflammation of the pancreas, often resulting in severe abdominal pain, nausea, vomiting, and potentially life-threatening complications.

Here are some strategies on coping with acute pancreatitis:

♥ Seek Medical Help:

If you suspect acute pancreatitis, it's crucial to seek medical attention promptly. Symptoms often require urgent evaluation in an emergency room or by a healthcare professional. Treatment may involve hospitalization, pain management, intravenous fluids to prevent dehydration, and addressing potential complications.

♥ NPO (Nil Per Os):

In the initial phase of acute pancreatitis, the digestive system may need a break to allow the pancreas to heal. This typically involves a period of fasting where no food or drink is consumed to reduce the workload on the pancreas and decrease stimulation of digestive enzymes. This is usually followed by a gradual reintroduction of food as recommended by the healthcare provider.

♥ Pain Management:

Acute pancreatitis often causes severe abdominal pain. Pain relief is vital and may involve medication prescribed by a healthcare professional. Nonsteroidal anti-inflammatory drugs (NSAIDs) are generally avoided due to the risk of exacerbating the condition.

♥ Fluid Intake:

Hydration is essential to prevent complications like dehydration. Intravenous fluids are commonly administered to maintain adequate hydration levels and support the body during recovery.

♥ Nutritional Support:

As the patient's condition improves, a gradual reintroduction of food occurs. The specific diet plan during recovery may vary based on the severity of the pancreatitis and individual needs. Generally, a low-fat diet is recommended to ease the workload on the pancreas and reduce the risk of triggering further inflammation.

♥ Avoid Alcohol:

Alcohol consumption is a common cause of pancreatitis. To prevent recurrence, it's crucial to abstain from alcohol completely.

♥ Follow-up Care:

After discharge, regular follow-up visits with healthcare providers are important to monitor recovery, assess nutritional needs, and address any ongoing concerns or complications.

Adopting a healthy lifestyle by maintaining a balanced diet, regular exercise, and avoiding triggers such as excessive alcohol consumption or high-fat foods can help prevent future episodes of pancreatitis.

Addressing the complexities of chronic pancreatitis

Chronic pancreatitis is a state characterized by inflammation of the pancreas that persists over time, leading to long-term damage to this important organ. Managing chronic pancreatitis involves a multi-faceted approach that includes dietary changes, lifestyle modifications, and medical treatment.

Understanding Chronic Pancreatitis

Chronic pancreatitis takes place when the pancreas becomes inflamed and this inflammation doesn't improve, causing lasting damage. The pancreas, crucial for digestion and hormone regulation, gets affected, leading to difficulties in properly digesting food and regulating blood sugar levels.

Tackling Chronic Pancreatitis through Diet

✓ **Low-Fat Diet:**

Reduce fat intake as it can trigger pancreatic enzyme production, leading to discomfort. Focus on lean proteins, fruits, vegetables, and whole grains while minimizing fried foods, fatty meats, and high-fat dairy.

✓ **Small, Frequent Meals:**

Eating short meals throughout the day helps reduce stress on the pancreas, aiding in better digestion and absorption of nutrients.

✓ **Limited Alcohol and Caffeine:**

Alcohol and caffeine can exacerbate pancreatitis. Avoiding or minimizing their intake can alleviate symptoms and reduce the risk of complications.

✓ **Hydration and Balanced Nutrition:**

Staying hydrated and maintaining a balanced diet rich in nutrients, including vitamins A, C, D, and E, is essential. Supplements might be necessary if deficiencies are present.

✓ **Enzyme Replacement Therapy:**

Some individuals might require pancreatic enzyme supplements to aid digestion, especially when the pancreas isn't producing sufficient enzymes.

✓ **Avoid Catalyst Foods:**

Certain foods, such as spicy, greasy, and processed foods, can aggravate symptoms. Identifying and avoiding these triggers is crucial.

✓ **Consult a Registered Dietitian or Nutritionist:**

Personalized dietary plans are crucial for managing chronic pancreatitis. Consulting a professional can help create a diet tailored to individual needs.

Nutritional Do's and Don'ts for pancreatic well-being

When considering a diet for pancreatic health, it's essential to focus on foods that support healing and reduce inflammation while avoiding those that may exacerbate pancreatitis. Here's a breakdown of Nutritional Do's and Don'ts for pancreatic well-being:

Do's:

⮕ **Low-Fat Foods:**

Opt for low-fat or fat-free versions of dairy, such as skim milk, low-fat yogurt, and cheese. Avoid high-fat foods like fried items, fatty cuts of meat, and full-fat dairy as they can trigger pancreatitis.

⮕ **Lean Protein:**

Choose lean types of protein like skinless poultry, fish, tofu, and legumes. These are easier for your pancreas to process compared to fatty meats.

⮕ **Complex Carbohydrates:**

Focus on whole grains like brown rice, whole wheat bread, quinoa, oats, and barley. They provide essential nutrients and fiber without causing spikes in blood sugar levels.

⮕ **Healthy Fats:**

Include healthy fats from sources like avocados, nuts, beans, and olive oil in moderation. These fats support overall health without putting stress on the pancreas.

⮕ **Fruits and Vegetables:**

Emphasize a variety of colorful fruits and vegetables as they are enriched in antioxidants and vitamins. However, avoid citrus fruits if they cause discomfort.

⮕ **Hydration:**

Drink plenty of water all through the day to stay hydrated and support digestion. Avoid sugary beverages and excessive caffeine.

Don'ts:

✷ **High-Fat Foods:**

Stay away from fried foods, fatty cuts of meat, processed foods, and high-fat dairy products. These can trigger inflammation and worsen pancreatitis symptoms.

✷ **Sugary Foods:**

Limit intake of sugary snacks, desserts, and beverages as they can spike blood sugar levels and stress the pancreas.

✷ **Alcohol:**

Avoid or limit alcohol consumption as it can inflame the pancreas and lead to pancreatitis or worsen existing conditions.

✷ **Trans Fats and Processed Foods:**

Steer clear of foods containing trans fats, hydrogenated oils, and heavily processed items like fast food, packaged snacks, and pastries.

✷ **Spicy and Greasy Foods:**

These can irritate the digestive system and worsen symptoms. Avoid spicy dishes and greasy foods like pizza or heavily sauced meals.

✷ **Caffeine:**

While moderate caffeine intake may be okay for some, it's wise to limit or avoid it if it tends to trigger discomfort or exacerbate symptoms.

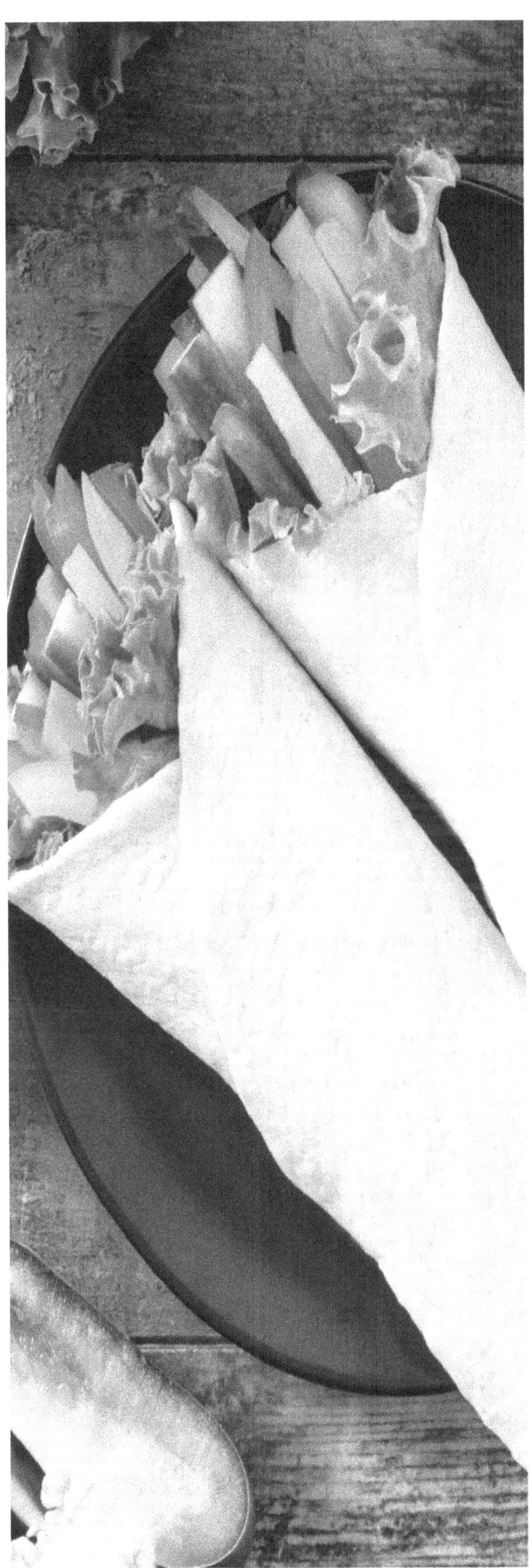

Oatmeal with Blueberries

Serving: 1-2

Prep Time: 5 minutes

Cook Time: 10 minutes

Ingredients:

- 1 cup rolled oats
- 2 cups water
- 1/2 cup fresh blueberries
- 1 tablespoon honey (optional)
- Cinnamon (optional)

Directions:

1. In a saucepan, bring water to a boil.
2. Spoon in rolled oats and reduce heat to a simmer. Cook for 5-7 minutes or until oats are tender, stirring occasionally.
3. Reduce from heat and let it cool slightly.
4. Add fresh blueberries on top and drizzle with honey if desired. Sprinkle with a dash of cinnamon for added flavor.

Nutrition Information (per serving):

Calories: 220, Carbohydrates: 45g, Protein: 5g, Fat: 3g, Fiber: 6g, Sugar: 10g

Banana Walnut Pancakes

Serving: 1-2

Prep Time: 10 minutes

Cook Time: 10 minutes

Ingredients:

- 1 ripe banana, mashed
- 1 cup oat flour (blend rolled oats to make flour)
- 1 teaspoon baking powder

- 1/2 cup milk (almond) (or any milk substitute)
- 1/4 cup chopped walnuts
- Cooking spray or a little oil for the pan

Directions:

Directions:

1. In a mixing bowl, combine mashed banana, oat flour, baking powder, and almond milk. Mix until well combined. Fold in chopped walnuts.
2. Heat up a non-stick fry pan over medium heat and slightly coat with cooking spray or oil.
3. Lay 1/4 cup of batter onto the skillet for each pancake. Stir until the bubbles form on the surface, then flip until golden brown on both sides.
4. Serve searing hot with a drizzle of honey or a dollop of yogurt if desired.

Nutrition Information (per serving):

Calories: 320, Carbohydrates: 45g, Protein: 8g, Fat: 12gFiber: 6g, Sugar: 12g

Egg White Veggie Omelette

Serving: 1-2

Prep Time: 7 minutes

Cook Time: 5 minutes

Ingredients:

- 4 egg whites
- 1/4 cup diced up bell peppers (any color)
- 1/4 cup diced onions
- 1/4 cup diced tomatoes
- Salt and pepper to taste
- 1 teaspoon olive oil

Directions:

1. Heat up the olive oil in a non-sticky skillet over medium heat.
2. Add diced bell peppers, onions, and tomatoes. Sauté for 2-3 minutes until vegetables are tender.
3. Whisk egg whites in a bowl and pour over the sautéed vegetables in the skillet.
4. Let the eggs cook for a few minutes until set. Season with salt and pepper.
5. Carefully wrap the omelette in half and slide it onto a plate.

Nutrition Information (per serving):

Calories: 120, Carbohydrates: 8g, Protein: 20g, Fat: 2g, Fiber: 2g, Sugar: 4g

Fruit Salad

Serving: 1-2

Prep Time: 10 minutes

Ingredients:

- 1 cup mixed fruits (such as diced apples, berries, grapes, and melon)
- 1 tablespoon lemon juice
- 1 tablespoon honey (optional)
- Fresh mint leaves for garnish (optional)

Directions:

1. In a mixing bowl, combine all the diced fruits.
2. Drizzle lemon juice over the fruits and gently toss to coat evenly. Add honey if desired for sweetness.
3. Garnish with fresh mint leaves before serving.

Nutrition Information (per serving):

Calories: 80, Carbohydrates: 20g, Protein: 1g, Fat: 0g, Fiber: 3g, Sugar: 15g

Serving: 1-2

Prep Time: 5 minutes

Ingredients:

- 1 cup Greek yogurt (low-fat or non-fat)
- 1/2 cup fresh berries (blueberries, strawberries, or raspberries)
- 1/4 cup granola (low-fat, low-sugar)
- 1 tablespoon honey (optional)

Directions:

1. Into a glass or bowl, layer Greek yogurt, berries, and granola.
2. Redo the layers until the glass or bowl is filled.
3. Drizzle with honey if desired.
4. Serve immediately.

Nutrition Information (per serving):

Calories: 200-250 kcal, Protein: 15-20g, Fat: 5-7g, Carbohydrates: 25-30g

Serving: 1-2

Prep Time: 5 minutes

Ingredients:

- 2 slices whole wheat bread
- 2 tablespoons almond butter (unsweetened)
- Cinnamon (optional)

Directions:

1. Toast the whole wheat bread slices.
2. Spread almond butter evenly on the toasted bread.
3. Sprinkle a dash of cinnamon for extra flavor if desired.
4. Serve immediately.

Nutrition Information (per serving):

Calories: 250-300 kcal, Protein: 8-10g, Fat: 12-15g, Carbohydrates: 30-35g

Serving: 1-2

Prep Time: 10 minutes

Cook Time: 15 minutes

Ingredients:

- 1/2 cup quinoa (rinsed)
- 1 cup water or low-sodium vegetable broth
- 1/2 cup chopped fruits (such as apples, berries, or bananas)
- 2 tablespoons chopped nuts (almonds, walnuts, or pecans)
- Cinnamon (optional)

Directions:

1. Into a saucepan, bring water or vegetable broth to a boil. Add quinoa and reduce heat to low.
2. Cover and simmer for 15 minutes or until quinoa is cooked and liquid is absorbed.
3. Mush the quinoa with a fork and then move it to a bowl.
4. Top with chopped fruits, nuts, and sprinkle with cinnamon if desired.
5. Serve warm.

Nutrition Information (per serving):

Calories: 300-350 kcal, Protein: 8-10g, Fat: 10-12g, Carbohydrates: 40-45g

Serving: 1-2

Prep Time: 5 minutes

Ingredients:

- 1 ripe banana
- 1/2 cup plain Greek yogurt (low-fat or non-fat)

- 1/2 cup fresh or canned berries (blueberries, strawberries, raspberries)
- 1/2 cup spinach or kale (washed)
- 1/2 cup unsweetened milk or water
- 1 tablespoon honey (optional)

Directions:

1. Combine all ingredients in a blender.
2. Blend until smooth and creamy.
3. Add honey if desired for sweetness.
4. Pour into a glass and serve immediately.

Nutrition Information (per serving):

Calories: 200-250 kcal, Protein: 8-10g, Fat: 3-5g, Carbohydrates: 35-40g

Cottage Cheese with Pineapple

Serving: 1-2

Prep Time: 5 minutes

Ingredients:

- 1 cup low-fat cottage cheese
- 1/2 cup diced pineapple (fresh or canned in juice)

Directions:

1. In a bowl, combine cottage cheese and diced pineapple.
2. Mix gently.
3. Serve immediately.

Nutrition Information (per serving):

Calories: 150-200 kcal, Protein: 15-20g, Fat: 2-4g, Carbohydrates: 15-20g

Baked Apple with Cinnamon

Serving: 1-2

Prep Time: 5 minutes

Cook Time: 25 minutes

Ingredients:

- 1 apple
- 1/2 teaspoon cinnamon
- 1 teaspoon honey (optional)
- 1 tablespoon chopped walnuts (optional)

Directions:

1. Put your oven on 350°F (175°C).
2. Wash the apple thoroughly and remove the core, creating a hollow in the center but leaving the bottom intact to hold the filling.
3. Place the apple in a baking dish.
4. Sprinkle the cinnamon evenly over the apple. If desired, drizzle honey over the top for added sweetness.
5. Optionally, stuff the hollowed center with chopped walnuts.
6. Bake in the oven for about 25 minutes or until the apple is tender and lightly browned.

Nutrition Information (per serving, without optional honey and walnuts):

Calories: 95, Carbohydrates: 25g, Fiber: 4g, Sugar: 19g, Fat: 0g, Protein: 0g

Avocado Toast

Serving: 1-2

Prep Time: 5 minutes

Cook Time: 5 minutes

Ingredients:

- 1 ripe avocado
- 2 slices of whole grain bread
- 1 tablespoon lemon juice
- Salt and pepper to taste
- Optional: Red pepper flakes, cherry tomatoes (for garnish)

Directions:

1. Carve up the avocado in half, take out the pit, and scoop out it into a bowl. Mash up the avocado with a fork.
2. Add up the lime juice, salt, and pepper to the mashed avocado. Mix until well combined.
3. Toast the pieces of whole grain bread until they reach your desired level of crispiness.
4. Spread the mashed avocado mixture evenly over the toasted bread slices.
5. Optionally, garnish with red pepper flakes or sliced cherry tomatoes for added flavor.

Calories: 220, Carbohydrates: 20g, Fiber: 10g, Sugar: 1g, Fat: 15g, Protein: 6g

Muesli with Low-Fat Milk

Servings: 1-2

Prep Time: 5 minutes

Ingredients:

- 1/2 cup rolled oats
- 1 tablespoon chopped almonds
- 1 tablespoon chopped walnuts
- 1 tablespoon ground flaxseeds
- 1/2 cup low-fat milk
- 1/2 teaspoon honey (optional)

Directions:

1. In a bowl, combine rolled oats, almonds, walnuts, and ground flaxseeds.
2. Pour in the low-fat milk and mix well. Add honey if desired.
3. Let it sit for a few minutes to allow the oats to soften slightly before enjoying.

Nutrition Information (per serving):

Calories: 250, Protein: 9g, Fat: 11g, Carbohydrates: 30g, Fiber: 6g

Veggie Breakfast Burrito

Servings: 1-2

Prep Time: 10 minutes

Cook Time: 10 minutes

Ingredients:

- 2 whole-grain tortillas
- 4 eggs (or egg substitute)
- 1/4 cup diced bell peppers
- 1/4 cup diced onions
- 1/4 cup chopped spinach
- Salt and pepper to taste

Directions:

1. In a non-stick skillet, sauté diced bell peppers, onions, and spinach until softened.
2. Whisk eggs and pour into the skillet with the veggies. Cook until the eggs are set.
3. Carve the egg and veggie mixture between the tortillas, roll them up, and serve.

Nutrition Information (per serving):

Calories: 300, Protein: 18g, Fat: 10g, Carbohydrates: 30g, Fiber: 5g

Rice Cake with Hummus

Servings: 1-2

Prep Time: 5 minutes

Ingredients:

- 2 rice cakes
- 4 tablespoons hummus (low-fat)
- Sliced cucumbers, tomatoes, or bell peppers (optional)

Directions:

1. Spread a generous layer of hummus onto each rice cake.
2. Top with sliced vegetables if desired.

Calories: 150, Protein: 4g, Fat: 6g, Carbohydrates: 20g, Fiber: 2g

Steamed Vegetables with Tofu

Servings: 1-2

Prep Time: 10 minutes

Cook Time: 10 minutes

Ingredients:

- Assorted vegetables (broccoli, carrots, bell peppers, etc.)
- 6 ounces tofu (firm or extra firm), cubed
- Low-sodium vegetable broth or water
- Herbs and spices of choice (optional)

Directions:

1. Cut vegetables into bite-sized pieces.
2. Steam vegetables until slightly tender.
3. In a separate pan, lightly sauté tofu cubes with herbs and spices.
4. Serve steamed vegetables with tofu on the side.

Nutrition Information (per serving):

Calories: 200, Protein: 14g, Fat: 8g, Carbohydrates: 18g, Fiber: 6g

Chia Seed Pudding

Servings: 1-2

Prep Time: 5 minutes (+ refrigeration time)

Ingredients:

- 1/4 cup chia seeds
- 1 cup low-fat milk
- 1/2 teaspoon vanilla extract
- 1 tablespoon honey or maple syrup (optional)

Directions:

1. In a bowl or jar, mix chia seeds, low-fat milk, vanilla extract, and sweetener if desired.
2. Stir well and refrigerate for at least 2 hours or overnight until it thickens.
3. Serve chilled, topped with fresh fruits or nuts if desired.

Nutrition Information (per serving):

Calories: 180, Protein: 7g, Fat: 8g, Carbohydrates: 20g, Fiber: 10g

Whole Grain Waffles with Berries

Servings: 2-3

Prep Time: 10 minutes

Cook Time: 10 minutes

Ingredients:

- 1 cup whole grain waffle mix
- 1 egg (or egg substitute)
- ¾ cup low-fat milk
- 1 tablespoon vegetable oil
- ½ cup mixed berries (blueberries, strawberries, raspberries)
- 1 tablespoon honey or maple syrup (optional)

Directions:

1. Set the waffle iron according to manufacturer's instructions.

2. Into a mixing bowl, combine the waffle mix, egg, milk, and vegetable oil. Mix until just combined.
3. Lay the batter onto the preheated waffle iron and cook until golden brown and crisp.
4. Top the waffles with mixed berries and drizzle with honey or maple syrup if desired.

Calories: 250, Total Fat: 8g, Saturated Fat: 1.5g, Cholesterol: 55mg, Sodium: 350mg, Total Carbohydrates: 38g, Dietary Fiber: 5g, Sugars: 10g, Protein: 8g

Brown Rice Porridge

Servings: 1-2

Prep Time: 5 minutes

Cook Time: 25 minutes

Ingredients:

- 1 cup cooked brown rice
- 1 ½ cups low-fat milk or almond milk
- 1 tablespoon honey or maple syrup
- ½ teaspoon ground cinnamon
- ¼ cup chopped nuts (almonds, walnuts) for garnish (optional)

Directions:

1. In a saucepan, combine the cooked brown rice, milk, honey or maple syrup, and ground cinnamon.
2. Bring the compound to a gentle simmer over medium-low heat, stirring occasionally.
3. Cook for 20-25 minutes or until the porridge thickens to your desired consistency, stirring occasionally.
4. Serve warm, garnished with chopped nuts if desired.

Nutrition Information (per serving):

Calories: 300, Total Fat: 8g, Saturated Fat: 1g, Cholesterol: 5mg, Sodium: 100mg, Total Carbohydrates: 50g, Dietary Fiber: 3g, Sugars: 15g, Protein: 7g

Spinach and Feta Frittata

Servings: 2-3

Prep Time: 10 minutes

Cook Time: 20 minutes

Ingredients:

- 4 large eggs
- ½ cup chopped spinach
- ¼ cup crumbled feta cheese
- 2 tablespoons low-fat milk or almond milk
- Salt and pepper to taste
- 1 teaspoon olive oil

Directions:

1. Adjust the oven temperature to 350°F (175°C).
2. In a mixing bowl, beat the eggs. Add the chopped spinach, feta cheese, milk, salt, and pepper. Mix well.
3. Put the olive oil in an oven-safe skillet on medium.
4. Lay the egg mixture into the skillet and cook for 3-4 minutes or until the edges start to set.
5. Remove the skillet to the preheated oven and cook it for 12-15 minutes until the frittata is set and slightly golden on top.
6. Slice and serve warm.

Nutrition Information (per serving):

Calories: 180, Total Fat: 12g, Saturated Fat: 4g, Cholesterol: 260mg, Sodium: 350mg, Total Carbohydrates: 3g, Dietary Fiber: 1g, Sugars: 1g, Protein: 14g

Servings: 6

Prep Time: 15 minutes

Cook Time: 20 minutes

Ingredients:

- 1 cup oat bran
- ½ cup whole wheat flour
- ½ teaspoon baking soda
- 1 teaspoon baking powder
- ½ teaspoon ground cinnamon
- ¼ cup unsweetened applesauce
- ¼ cup honey or maple syrup
- 1 egg
- ½ cup low-fat milk or almond milk
- ¼ cup raisins or chopped nuts (optional)

Directions:

1. The oven should be 375°F (190°C).Grease or lay a muffin tin with liners.
2. In a mixing bowl, combine oat bran, whole wheat flour, baking soda, baking powder, and ground cinnamon.
3. In another bowl, whisk together applesauce, honey or maple syrup, egg, and milk.
4. Lay the liquid ingredients into the dry ingredients and stir until just combined. Fold in raisins or nuts if using.
5. Separate the batter evenly into the prepared muffin tin.
6. Cook it for 18-20 minutes or until a toothpick inserted into the inside comes out clean.
7. Allow muffins to cool before serving.

Nutrition Information (per serving - 1 muffin):

Calories: 140, Total Fat: 2g, Saturated Fat: 0.5g, Cholesterol: 25mg, Sodium: 150mg, Total Carbohydrates: 29g, Dietary Fiber: 4g, Sugars: 12g, Protein: 5g

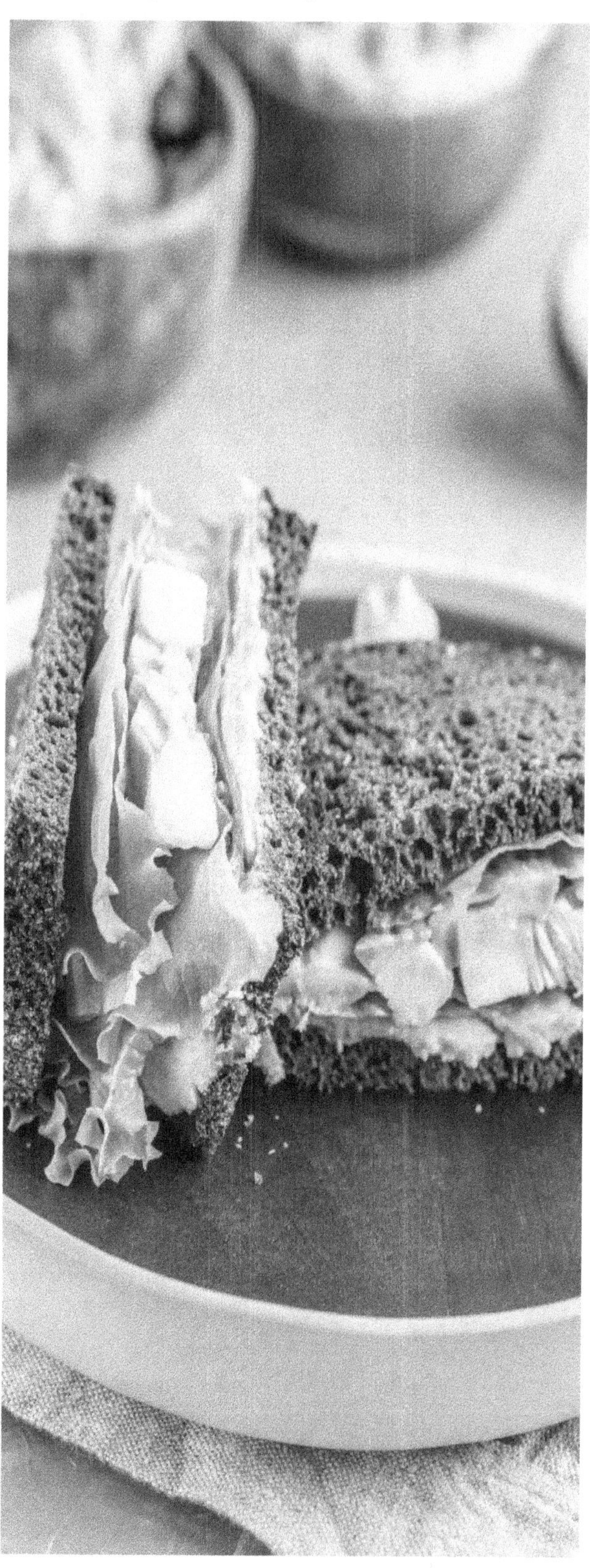

Grilled Vegetable Salad

Serving: 2

Prep Time: 15 minutes

Cook Time: 10 minutes

Ingredients:

- 2 cups mixed vegetables (zucchini, bell peppers, eggplant, etc.)
- 2 cups mixed greens (spinach, kale, arugula)
- 2 tablespoons olive oil
- Salt and pepper to taste
- 2 tablespoons balsamic vinegar

Directions:

1. Preset a grill or grill pan over medium heat.
2. Cut the vegetables into bite-sized pieces.
3. Saute the vegetables with olive oil, salt, and pepper.
4. Sear the vegetables for about 5 minutes on each side until they are tender and have grill marks.
5. In a bowl, mix the grilled vegetables with mixed greens.
6. Dribble balsamic vinegar over the salad and toss gently to combine.
7. Serve immediately.

Nutrition Information (per serving):

Calories: 180, Total Fat: 10g, Carbohydrates: 20g, Fiber: 7g, Protein: 5g

Quinoa and Black Bean Salad

Serving: 2

Prep Time: 15 minutes

Cook Time: 15 minutes

Ingredients:

- 1 cup cooked quinoa
- 1 cup black beans (canned, drained, and rinsed)
- 1 red bell pepper, diced
- 1/4 cup chopped cilantro
- 2 tablespoons lime juice
- 2 tablespoons olive oil
- Salt and pepper to taste

Directions:

1. In a bowl, combine cooked quinoa, black beans, diced bell pepper, and chopped cilantro.
2. Take a separate small bowl, whisk together lime juice, olive oil, salt, and pepper.
3. Spread the dressing over the quinoa mixture and toss gently to coat evenly.
4. Cool it in the refrigerator for at least 30 minutes before serving.
5. Serve chilled.

Nutrition Information (per serving):

Calories: 320, Total Fat: 12g, Carbohydrates: 45g, Fiber: 12g, Protein: 12g

Miso Soup with Tofu and Vegetables

Serving: 2

Prep Time: 10 minutes

Cook Time: 10 minutes

Ingredients:

- 4 cups water
- 2 tablespoons miso paste
- 1 cup tofu, cubed
- 1 cup sliced mushrooms
- 1 cup chopped spinach or bok choy
- 2 green onions, sliced
- 1 teaspoon sesame oil (optional)

Directions:

1. Into a pot, bring water to a gentle boil.
2. Decrease heat to low and whisk in miso paste until dissolved.
3. Add tofu, mushrooms, and greens to the pot.
4. Simmer for about 5-7 minutes until the vegetables are tender.
5. Stir in sliced green onions and sesame oil (if using) just before serving.
6. Serve hot.

Nutrition Information (per serving):

Calories: 120, Total Fat: 6g, Carbohydrates: 8g, Fiber: 2g, Protein: 10g

Turkey and Veggie Wrap

Serving: 1

Prep Time: 10 minutes

Ingredients:

- 1 large whole wheat or gluten-free wrap
- 3 ounces sliced turkey breast
- 1/2 cup shredded lettuce
- 1/4 cup sliced cucumber
- 1/4 cup sliced bell peppers
- 2 tablespoons hummus

Directions:

1. Spread the wrap flat on a clean surface.
2. Spread hummus evenly over the wrap.
3. Layer sliced turkey, shredded lettuce, sliced cucumber, and bell peppers on top of the hummus.
4. Wrap in the sides of the wrap and roll it tightly.
5. Slice in half diagonally if desired.
6. Set out immediately or wrap in foil for later.

Nutrition Information (per serving):

Calories: 300, Total Fat: 8g, Carbohydrates: 30g, Fiber: 7g, Protein: 25g

Tuna Salad Lettuce Wraps

Servings: 1-2

Prep Time: 15 minutes

Cook Time: 0 minutes

Ingredients:

- 1 can (5 oz) tuna in water, drained
- 2 tablespoons plain Greek yogurt
- 1 tablespoon finely chopped celery
- 1 tablespoon finely chopped red onion
- 1 tablespoon chopped fresh parsley
- Salt and pepper to taste
- 4 large lettuce leaves (such as romaine or iceberg)
- Optional: Sliced cucumber or avocado for garnish

Directions:

1. Take a mixing bowl, combine the drained tuna, Greek yogurt, celery, red onion, parsley, salt, and pepper. Mix until well combined.
2. Lay out the lettuce leaves on a clean surface. Spoon the tuna salad mixture evenly onto each lettuce leaf.
3. Optionally, add slices of cucumber or avocado on top of the tuna salad.
4. Roll up the lettuce leaves like a wrap, enclosing the filling.
5. Plate out immediately or refrigerate until ready to eat.

Nutrition Information (per serving):

Calories: 160, Protein: 20g, Fat: 3g, Carbohydrates: 8g, Fiber: 2g

Servings: 2

Prep Time: 10 minutes

Cook Time: 20 minutes

Ingredients:

- 1 cup cooked brown rice
- 1 tablespoon olive oil
- 1 cup mixed vegetables (bell peppers, broccoli, carrots, snap peas)
- 1/2 cup diced cooked chicken or tofu (optional)
- 2 tablespoons low-sodium soy sauce
- 1 teaspoon minced ginger
- 1 clove garlic, minced
- Salt and pepper to taste
- Chopped green onions for garnish

Directions:

1. Put in olive oil in a skillet over medium-high heat. Add minced ginger and garlic, stir for 30 seconds.
2. Include mixed vegetables to the skillet and stir-fry for 3-4 minutes until slightly tender.
3. Add diced chicken or tofu (if using) and cooked brown rice to the skillet. Stir well to combine.
4. Pour in the low-sodium soy sauce and continue cooking for an additional 2-3 minutes.
5. Season with salt and pepper to taste.
6. Garnish with chopped green onions before serving.

Nutrition Information (per serving):

Calories: 280, Protein: 12g, Fat: 8g, Carbohydrates: 40g, Fiber: 5g

Servings: 4

Prep Time: 10 minutes

Cook Time: 30 minutes

Ingredients:

- 1 cup dry green or red lentils, rinsed
- 4 cups low-sodium vegetable broth
- 1 tablespoon olive oil
- 1 onion, chopped
- 2 carrots, diced
- 2 celery stalks, diced
- 2 cloves garlic, minced
- 1 teaspoon ground cumin
- 1 teaspoon paprika
- Salt and pepper to taste
- Fresh parsley for garnish

Directions:

1. Take a large pot, heat olive oil over medium heat. Add chopped onion, carrots, celery, and minced garlic. Sauté for 5 minutes until vegetables are slightly softened.
2. Add lentils, vegetable broth, ground cumin, paprika, salt, and pepper to the pot. Stir well.
3. Bring the soup to a boil, then reduce heat to low and let it simmer for 20-25 minutes until lentils are tender.
4. Adjust seasoning if needed and serve hot, garnished with fresh parsley.

Nutrition Information (per serving):

Calories: 220, Protein: 13g, Fat: 4g, Carbohydrates: 34g, Fiber: 12g

Hummus and Veggie Sandwich

Servings: 2

Prep Time: 10 minutes

Cook Time: 0 minutes

Ingredients:

- 4 slices whole grain bread
- 1/2 cup hummus (store-bought or homemade)
- 1 cucumber, thinly sliced
- 1 large tomato, thinly sliced
- 1 cup baby spinach leaves
- Optional: Sprouts or shredded carrots for extra crunch

Directions:

1. Toast the slices of whole grain bread if desired.
2. Spread a generous amount of hummus on each slice of bread.
3. Layer cucumber slices, tomato slices, and baby spinach leaves on two slices of bread.
4. Optionally, add sprouts or shredded carrots for extra texture.
5. Season with the remaining slices of bread to make sandwiches.
6. Slice the sandwiches in half if desired and serve immediately.

Nutrition Information (per serving):

Calories: 320, Protein: 12g, Fat: 10g, Carbohydrates: 48g, Fiber: 10g

Caprese Salad

Servings: 1-2

Prep Time: 10 minutes

Ingredients:

- 2 medium tomatoes, sliced
- 1 cup fresh mozzarella cheese, sliced
- Fresh basil leaves

- 2 tablespoons extra virgin olive oil
- Salt and pepper to taste

Directions:

1. Arrange tomato and mozzarella slices on a plate.
2. Tuck basil leaves in between slices.
3. Drizzle with olive oil.
4. Season with salt and pepper.
5. Serve fresh.

Nutrition Information (per serving):

Calories: 250, Protein: 12g, Fat: 20g, Carbohydrates: 5g

Sweet Potato and Chickpea Salad

Servings: 2

Prep Time: 15 minutes

Cook Time: 20 minutes

Ingredients:

- 2 medium sweet potatoes, peeled and cubed
- 1 can (15 oz) chickpeas, drained off and rinsed
- 2 tablespoons olive oil
- 1 teaspoon paprika
- Salt and pepper to taste
- Fresh parsley for garnish (optional)

Directions:

1. Preheat oven to 400°F (200°C).
2. Toss sweet potatoes and chickpeas with olive oil, paprika, salt, and pepper.
3. Roll out on a baking sheet and roast for 20 minutes or until tender.
4. Let it cool slightly, garnish with parsley (if using), and serve.

Nutrition Information (per serving):

Calories: 350, Protein: 10g, Fat: 12g, Carbohydrates: 50g

Zucchini Noodles with Marinara Sauce

Servings: 2

Prep Time: 15 minutes

Cook Time: 10 minutes

Ingredients:

- 2 medium zucchinis, spiralized
- 1 cup marinara sauce (low-fat and low-sugar)
- 2 tablespoons grated Parmesan cheese (optional)
- Fresh basil leaves for garnish

Directions:

1. In a pan, heat marinara sauce over medium heat.
2. Add zucchini noodles and cook for 5-7 minutes until tender.
3. Divide into plates, sprinkle with Parmesan cheese (if using), and garnish with basil leaves.

Nutrition Information (per serving):

Calories: 120, Protein: 5g, Fat: 3g, Carbohydrates: 20g

Broccoli and Cauliflower Soup

Servings: 2

Prep Time: 10 minutes

Cook Time: 20 minutes

Ingredients:

- 2 cups broccoli florets
- 2 cups cauliflower florets
- 1 onion, chopped
- 2 cloves garlic, minced
- 3 cups low-sodium vegetable broth
- Salt and pepper to taste

Directions:

1. In a pot, sauté onion and garlic until fragrant.
2. Add broccoli, cauliflower, and vegetable broth. Bring to a boil.
3. Decrease the heat and simmer for 15-20 minutes until vegetables are tender.
4. Mix until smooth using an immersion blender or regular blender.
5. Season with salt and pepper, serve hot.

Nutrition Information (per serving):

Calories: 120, Protein: 5g, Fat: 2g, Carbohydrates: 25g

Egg Salad Lettuce Wraps

Servings: 2

Prep Time: 10 minutes

Ingredients:

- 4 hard-boiled eggs, chopped
- 2 tablespoons plain Greek yogurt
- 1 tablespoon Dijon mustard
- 2 tablespoons chopped green onions
- Salt and pepper to taste
- Lettuce leaves for wrapping

Directions:

1. In a bowl, mix chopped eggs, Greek yogurt, mustard, green onions, salt, and pepper.
2. Spoon the egg salad onto lettuce leaves.
3. Wrap and serve.

Nutrition Information (per serving):

Calories: 180, Protein: 14g, Fat: 11g, Carbohydrates: 5g

Serving: 4 servings

Prep Time: 15 minutes

Cook Time: 40 minutes

Ingredients:

- 1 pre-made pie crust (store-bought or homemade)
- 4 large eggs
- 1 cup low-fat milk or lactose-free milk
- 1 cup diced mixed vegetables (bell peppers, spinach, tomatoes, etc.)
- 1/2 cup shredded low-fat cheese
- Salt and pepper to taste

Directions:

1. Preheat oven to 375°F (190°C).
2. Put the pie crust in a pie dish and press it down.
3. Take a bowl, whisk together eggs, milk, salt, and pepper.
4. Spread diced vegetables evenly in the pie crust.
5. Pour the egg mixture over the vegetables.
6. Sprinkle shredded cheese on top.
7. Bake for 35-40 minutes or until the quiche is set and lightly golden.
8. Allow it to cool for a few minutes before slicing.

Nutrition Information (per serving):

Calories: 250, Total Fat: 12g, Saturated Fat: 4g, Cholesterol: 190mg, Sodium: 380mg, Total Carbohydrates: 22g, Protein: 13g

Brown Rice and Bean Burrito Bowl

Serving: 2 servings

Prep Time: 10 minutes

Cook Time: 20 minutes

Ingredients:

- 1 cup cooked brown rice
- 1 cup tinned black beans (rinsed and drained)
- 1/2 cup diced tomatoes
- 1/4 cup diced red onion
- 1/2 avocado, sliced
- 1/4 cup chopped cilantro
- Juice of 1 lime
- Salt and pepper to taste

Directions:

1. In a bowl, mix together cooked brown rice and black beans.
2. Add diced tomatoes, red onion, avocado slices, and chopped cilantro.
3. Squeeze out lime juice over the mixture and season with salt and pepper.
4. Toss everything together gently.
5. Serve in bowls and enjoy.

Nutrition Information (per serving):

Calories: 380, Total Fat: 12g, Saturated Fat: 2g, Cholesterol: 0mg, Sodium: 300mg, Total Carbohydrates: 58g, Protein: 12g

Greek Salad with Grilled Chicken

Serving: 2 servings

Prep Time: 15 minutes

Cook Time: 15 minutes

Ingredients:

- 2 boneless, skinless chicken breasts
- 2 tablespoons olive oil
- 1 teaspoon dried oregano
- Salt and pepper to taste
- 4 cups mixed salad greens
- 1 cup cherry tomatoes, halved
- 1/2 cucumber, sliced
- 1/4 cup sliced red onion
- 1/4 cup crumbled feta cheese
- 2 tablespoons lemon juice
- 1 tablespoon red wine vinegar

1. Preset the grill or grill pan over medium-high heat.
2. Rub chicken breasts with olive oil, dried oregano, salt, and pepper.
3. Roast the chicken for 6-7 minutes per side or until fully cooked.
4. In a large bowl, combine salad greens, cherry tomatoes, cucumber, red onion, and feta cheese.
5. Into a small bowl, whisk together lemon juice, red wine vinegar, and one tablespoon of olive oil to make the dressing.
6. Slice grilled chicken and add it to the salad.
7. Dribble the dressing over the salad, toss gently, and serve.

Nutrition Information (per serving):

Calories: 320, Total Fat: 18g, Saturated Fat: 5g, Cholesterol: 90mg, Sodium: 380mg, Total Carbohydrates: 10g, Protein: 30g

Cauliflower Rice Stir-Fry

Serving: 2 servings

Prep Time: 10 minutes

Cook Time: 15 minutes

Ingredients:

- 1 small head cauliflower, grated or processed into "rice"
- 2 tablespoons olive oil
- 2 cloves garlic, minced
- 1 cup mixed vegetables (bell peppers, broccoli, carrots, etc.)
- 1 cup cooked diced chicken or tofu (optional)
- 2 tablespoons low-sodium soy sauce or tamari
- 1 teaspoon sesame oil (optional)
- Salt and pepper to taste

- Chopped green onions for garnish

Directions:

1. Put in olive oil in a large skillet or wok over medium heat.
2. Add minced garlic and sauté for a minute until fragrant.
3. Stir in mixed vegetables and cook for 3-4 minutes until slightly tender.
4. Add cauliflower rice and cooked chicken or tofu if using. Cook for another 5-6 minutes, stirring frequently.
5. Pour soy sauce and sesame oil (if using) over the mixture. Season with salt and pepper.
6. Cook for 2-3 minutes more, ensuring everything is heated through.
7. Garnish with chopped green onions and serve.

Nutrition Information (per serving, without chicken/tofu):

Calories: 120, Total Fat: 7g, Saturated Fat: 1g, Cholesterol: 0mg, Sodium: 580mg, Total Carbohydrates: 12g, Protein: 4g

Salmon Salad

Servings: 2

Prep Time: 15 minutes

Cook Time: 10 minutes

Ingredients:

- 2 salmon fillets (4-6 ounces each)
- 4 cups mixed salad greens
- 1 cucumber, sliced
- 1 cup cherry tomatoes, halved
- ¼ cup red onion, thinly sliced
- 2 tablespoons olive oil
- 1 tablespoon lemon juice
- Salt and pepper to taste

Directions:

1. Preset the oven to 375°F (190°C). Lay the salmon fillets on a baking paper lined with parchment paper.
2. Season with salt and pepper. Bake for 10 minutes or till the salmon is cooked through.
3. Into a large mixing bowl, combine the salad greens, cucumber, cherry tomatoes, and red onion.
4. Into a small bowl, whip together olive oil, lime juice, salt, & pepper to make the seasoning.
5. Once the salmon is cooked, let it cool slightly, then flake it into bite-sized pieces.
6. Add the flaked salmon to the salad. Dribble the dressing over the salad and toss gently to combine.
7. Serve the salmon salad immediately and enjoy!

<u>**Nutrition Information (per serving):**</u>

Calories: 320, Total Fat: 18g, Saturated Fat: 3g, Cholesterol: 70mg, Sodium: 180mg, Total Carbohydrate: 10g, Dietary Fiber: 3g, Sugars: 4g, Protein: 30g

Tofu Lettuce Wraps

Servings: 2

Prep Time: 20 minutes

Cook Time: 10 minutes

<u>**Ingredients:**</u>

- 1 block (14-16 ounces) firm tofu, drained and diced
- 2 tablespoons low-sodium soy sauce
- 1 tablespoon sesame oil
- 1 tablespoon rice vinegar
- 1 teaspoon honey or agave syrup
- 1 garlic clove, minced
- ½ teaspoon ground ginger
- 1 bell pepper, diced
- 1 carrot, grated
- 4-6 large lettuce leaves (such as butter or iceberg)
- Optional: shredded green onions and sesame seeds for garnish

<u>**Directions:**</u>

1. Take a bowl, mix together the soy sauce, sesame oil, rice vinegar, honey, minced garlic, and ground ginger to make the marinade.
2. Put in the diced tofu to the marinade and let it sit for about 10 minutes.
3. Heat a non-stick skillet over medium heat. Add the marinated tofu and cook for 5-7 minutes until tofu is slightly browned.
4. Add diced bell pepper and grated carrot to the skillet with tofu. Stir-fry for an additional 3-4 minutes until vegetables are tender yet crisp.
5. Spoon the tofu and vegetable mixture into lettuce leaves, creating wraps.
6. Season with chopped green onions and sesame seeds if desired.
7. Serve the tofu lettuce wraps immediately and enjoy!

<u>**Nutrition Information (per serving):**</u>

Calories: 230, Total Fat: 14g, Saturated Fat: 2g, Cholesterol: 0mg, Sodium: 420mg, Total Carbohydrate: 15g, Dietary Fiber: 4g, Sugars: 6g, Protein: 16g

Vegetable Pasta Primavera

Servings: 2

Prep Time: 15 minutes

Cook Time: 15 minutes

<u>**Ingredients:**</u>

- 6 ounces whole grain pasta
- 1 tablespoon olive oil
- 2 cloves garlic, minced

- 1 cup broccoli florets
- 1 cup sliced bell peppers (assorted colors)
- 1 cup sliced zucchini
- ½ cup cherry tomatoes, halved
- 2 tablespoons chopped fresh basil
- Salt and pepper to taste
- Grated Parmesan cheese (optional)

Directions:

1. Cook the pasta according to package instructions. Drain and set aside.
2. Put in olive oil in a large skillet over medium heat. Add minced garlic and sauté for 1 minute.
3. Add broccoli florets, sliced bell peppers, and sliced zucchini to the skillet. Sauté for 5-7 minutes until vegetables are tender-crisp.
4. Add the cooked pasta, cherry tomatoes, and chopped basil to the skillet. Toss everything together gently.
5. Season with salt and pepper to taste.
6. Optional: Sprinkle with grated Parmesan cheese before serving.
7. Serve the vegetable pasta primavera immediately and enjoy!

Nutrition Information (per serving):

Calories: 380, Total Fat: 10g, Saturated Fat: 1.5g, Cholesterol: 0mg, Sodium: 35mg, Total Carbohydrate: 62g, Dietary Fiber: 10g, Sugars: 8g, Protein: 14g

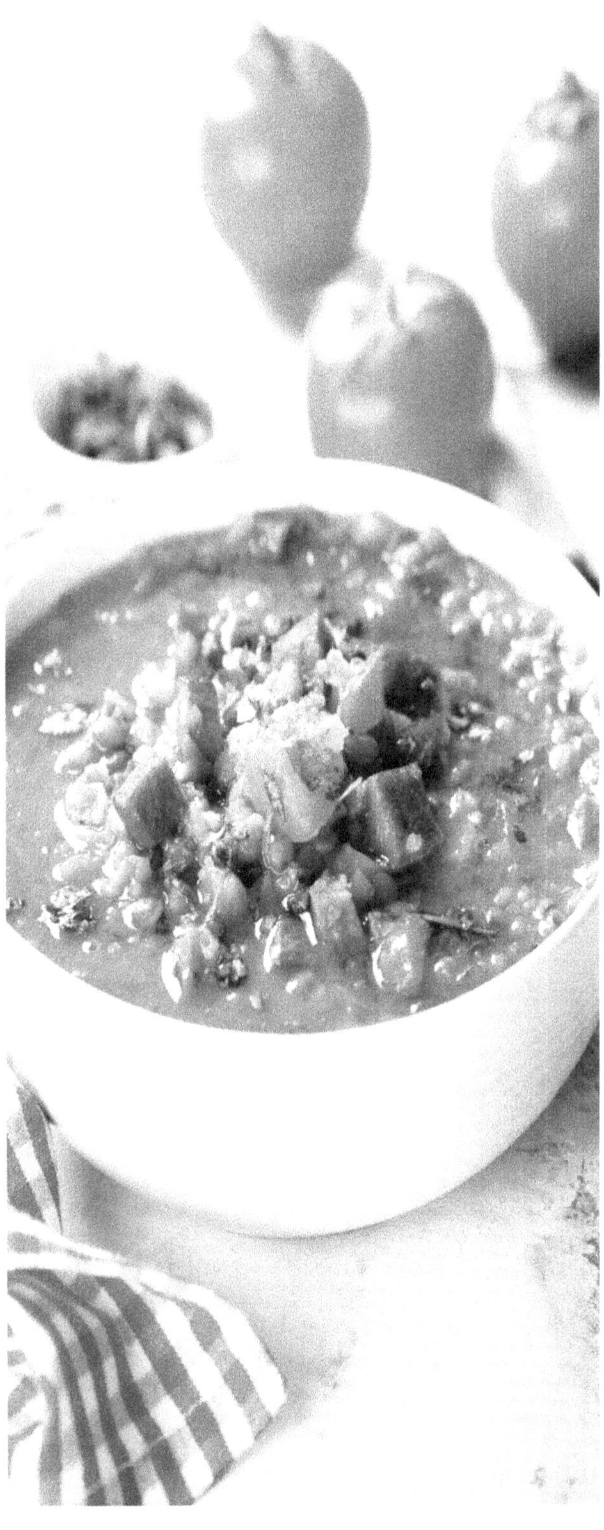

Baked Lemon Herb Chicken

Serving: 2

Prep Time: 10 minutes

Cook Time: 25 minutes

Ingredients:

- 2 boneless, skinless chicken breasts
- 2 tablespoons olive oil
- 2 tablespoons fresh lemon juice
- 1 teaspoon dried oregano
- 1 teaspoon dried thyme
- Salt and pepper to taste

Directions:

1. Put the oven on to 375°F (190°C).
2. Take a small bowl, mix olive oil, lemon juice, oregano, thyme, salt, and pepper.
3. Leave the chicken breasts in a baking dish and pour the herb mixture over them, coating evenly.
4. Bake for 25 minutes or until the chicken reaches an inward temperature of 165°F (74°C).
5. Set out with steamed vegetables or a side salad.

Nutrition Information (per serving):

Calories: 250, Protein: 30g, Fat: 12g, Carbohydrates: 2g, Fiber: 0.5g

Vegetable Stir-Fry with Tofu

Serving: 2

Prep Time: 15 minutes

Cook Time: 10 minutes

Ingredients:

- 1 block firm tofu, drained and cubed
- 2 cups mixed vegetables (bell peppers, broccoli, carrots, snap peas)
- 2 tablespoons low-sodium soy sauce
- 1 tablespoon sesame oil
- 1 teaspoon minced ginger
- 2 cloves garlic, minced
- 1 tablespoon olive oil
- Salt and pepper to taste

Directions:

1. Put the olive oil in a skillet over medium-high heat.
2. Add tofu cubes and stir-fry until lightly golden. Take out the tofu from the skillet and set aside.
3. In the same skillet, add sesame oil, ginger, and garlic. Cook for 30 seconds.
4. Add mixed vegetables and stir-fry for 5-7 minutes until tender yet crisp.
5. Return the tofu to the skillet, add soy sauce, and toss everything together for another 2 minutes.
6. Season with salt and pepper before serving.

Nutrition Information (per serving):

Calories: 280, Protein: 18g, Fat: 15g, Carbohydrates: 20g, Fiber: 6g

Salmon and Asparagus Foil Packets

Serving: 2

Prep Time: 10 minutes

Cook Time: 20 minutes

Ingredients:

- 2 salmon fillets
- 1 bunch asparagus, trimmed
- 2 tablespoons olive oil
- 2 cloves garlic, minced
- 1 teaspoon lemon zest
- Salt and pepper to taste

1. Put on the oven to 400°F (200°C).
2. Cut two large pieces of foil. Place each salmon fillet in the center of a piece of foil.
3. Divide the asparagus evenly between the foil packets, arranging them around the salmon.
4. Into a small bowl, mix olive oil, minced garlic, lemon zest, salt, and pepper. Drizzle this mixture over the salmon and asparagus.
5. Seal the foil packets tightly and place them on a baking sheet.
6. Bake for 18-20 minutes till the salmon is cooked through.
7. Serve with a side of brown rice or quinoa if desired.

Nutrition Information (per serving):

Calories: 320, Protein: 30g, Fat: 20g, Carbohydrates: 5g, Fiber: 3g

Mushroom and Spinach Pasta

Serving: 2

Prep Time: 10 minutes

Cook Time: 15 minutes

Ingredients:

- 6 oz whole wheat pasta
- 1 cup sliced mushrooms
- 2 cups fresh spinach
- 2 tablespoons olive oil
- 2 cloves garlic, minced
- 1 teaspoon dried basil
- Salt and pepper to taste

Directions:

1. Cook pasta according to package instructions. Drain and set aside.
2. Take a skillet, heat olive oil over medium heat. Add minced garlic and sauté for 30 seconds.
3. Add minsed mushrooms and cook for 5 minutes until they start to brown.
4. Adding up spinach to the skillet and cook until wilted.
5. Add the cooked pasta to the skillet, sprinkle with dried basil, salt, and pepper. Toss everything together for 2 minutes.
6. Serve hot.

Nutrition Information (per serving):

Calories: 350, Protein: 12g, Fat: 10g, Carbohydrates: 55g, Fiber: 8g

Roasted Vegetable and Quinoa Bowl

Serving: 2

Prep Time: 15 minutes

Cook Time: 25 minutes

Ingredients:

- 1 cup quinoa
- 2 cups mixed vegetables (bell peppers, zucchini, carrots)
- 2 tablespoons olive oil
- Salt and pepper to taste
- 1 teaspoon dry herbs (such as thyme or rosemary)

Directions:

1. Preheat oven to 400°F (200°C).
2. Cook quinoa according to package instructions.
3. Carve the vegetables into bite-sized pieces and place them on a baking sheet.
4. Dribble with olive oil, sprinkle with salt, pepper, and herbs. Toss to coat.
5. Bake in the oven for 20-25 minutes until the vegetables are tender and slightly golden.

6. Divide cooked quinoa into bowls, top with roasted vegetables, and serve.

Nutrition Information (per serving):

Calories: 350, Total Fat: 12g, Carbohydrates: 50g, Fiber: 8g, Protein: 10g

Black Bean and Corn Tacos

Serving: 2

Prep Time: 10 minutes

Cook Time: 10 minutes

Ingredients:

- 1 can (15 oz) black beans, drained off and rinsed
- 1 cup corn kernels
- 1 teaspoon olive oil
- 1 teaspoon chili powder
- Salt and pepper to taste
- 4 small corn tortillas
- Optional toppings: shredded lettuce, diced tomatoes, salsa

Directions:

1. Put on olive oil in a pan over medium heat. Add black beans, corn, chili powder, salt, and pepper. Cook for 5-7 minutes until heated through.
2. Warm the corn tortillas in a separate pan or microwave.
3. Split the bean and corn mixture among the tortillas.
4. Top with optional toppings if desired.
5. Serve immediately.

Nutrition Information (per serving):

Calories: 300, Total Fat: 4g, Carbohydrates: 60g, Fiber: 12g, Protein: 12g

Eggplant Parmesan

Serving: 2

Prep Time: 20 minutes

Cook Time: 25 minutes

Ingredients:

- 1 large eggplant, sliced into rounds
- 1 cup marinara sauce (low-fat, low-sodium)
- 1 cup breadcrumbs (whole wheat if available)
- 1/2 cup grated Parmesan cheese
- 1 teaspoon dried Italian herbs
- Olive oil spray

Directions:

1. Preheat oven to 400°F (200°C).
2. Dip eggplant slices in marinara sauce, then coat with breadcrumbs mixed with herbs and Parmesan cheese.
3. Lay the coated eggplant slices on a baking sheet lined with parchment paper.
4. Lightly spray with olive oil.
5. Bake for 20-25 minutes until slightly brown and crispy.
6. Serve warm.

Nutrition Information (per serving):

Calories: 280, Total Fat: 8g, Carbohydrates: 40g, Fiber: 10g, Protein: 12g

Veggie and Bean Chili

Serving: 4

Prep Time: 15 minutes

Cook Time: 30 minutes

Ingredients:

- 1 can (15 oz) kidney beans, drained and rinsed
- 1 can (15 oz) diced tomatoes

- 1 cup vegetable broth (low-sodium)
- 1 cup chopped mixed vegetables (bell peppers, onions, carrots)
- 1 teaspoon chili powder
- 1 teaspoon cumin
- Salt and pepper to taste

1. In a pot, combine diced tomatoes, kidney beans, mixed vegetables, vegetable broth, chili powder, cumin, salt, and pepper.
2. After a boil, then reduce heat and simmer for 20-25 minutes until vegetables are tender.
3. Adjust seasoning as needed.
4. Serve hot.

Nutrition Information (per serving):

Calories: 220, Total Fat: 1g, Carbohydrates: 45g, Fiber: 12g, Protein: 10g

Grilled Shrimp Skewers

Servings: 2

Prep Time: 15 minutes

Cook Time: 8 minutes

Ingredients:

- 12 large shrimp, peeled and deveined
- 1 tablespoon olive oil
- 1 clove garlic, minced
- 1 teaspoon lemon juice
- Salt and pepper to taste
- Skewers

Directions:

1. Preheat the grill to medium-high heat.
2. Take a bowl, combine olive oil, minced garlic, lemon juice, salt, and pepper. Add shrimp and toss to coat evenly.
3. Thread shrimp onto skewers.
4. Grill the skewers for about 4 minutes per side or until the shrimp turns pink and opaque.
5. Serve immediately and enjoy!

Nutrition Information (per serving):

Calories: 150, Protein: 18g, Fat: 7g, Carbohydrates: 2g, Fiber: 0g

Vegetable Curry

Servings: 2

Prep Time: 10 minutes

Cook Time: 20 minutes

Ingredients:

- 1 tablespoon olive oil
- 1 onion, finely chopped
- 2 cloves garlic, minced
- 1 teaspoon grated ginger
- 1 teaspoon curry powder
- 1 cup mixed vegetables (bell peppers, zucchini, carrots)
- 1 cup coconut milk
- Salt and pepper to taste

Directions:

1. Put on the olive oil in a pan over medium heat. Add chopped onion, garlic, and ginger. Sauté until fragrant.
2. Stir in curry powder and mixed vegetables. Cook for 5 minutes.
3. Add coconut milk, salt, and pepper. Simmer down for another 10 minutes until vegetables are tender.
4. Serve the vegetable curry over rice or with quinoa.

Nutrition Information (per serving):

Calories: 250, Protein: 4g, Fat: 20g, Carbohydrates: 15g, Fiber: 4g

Lentil and Vegetable Stew

Servings: 2

Prep Time: 10 minutes

Cook Time: 25 minutes

Ingredients:

- 1 tablespoon olive oil
- 1 onion, diced
- 2 carrots, sliced
- 2 celery stalks, chopped
- 1 cup dried lentils, rinsed
- 3 cups vegetable broth
- 1 bay leaf
- Salt and pepper to taste

Directions:

1. Put on olive oil in a pot over medium heat. Add diced onion, carrots, and celery. Sauté until softened.
2. Stir in dried lentils, vegetable broth, bay leaf, salt, and pepper. Bring to a boil.
3. Decrease heat, cover, and simmer for 20-25 minutes or until lentils are tender.
4. Remove bay leaf before serving. Enjoy this hearty lentil and vegetable stew!

Nutrition Information (per serving):

Calories: 320, Protein: 18g, Fat: 5g, Carbohydrates: 50g, Fiber: 20g

Cauliflower Steaks

Servings: 2

Prep Time: 10 minutes

Cook Time: 20 minutes

Ingredients:

- 1 large cauliflower head, leaves removed
- 2 tablespoons olive oil
- 1 teaspoon paprika
- Salt and pepper to taste

Directions:

1. Put on the oven to 400°F (200°C). Line a baking sheet with parchment paper.
2. Cut the cauliflower into 1-inch thick slices to make "steaks."
3. Into a small bowl, mix olive oil, paprika, salt, and pepper. Brush the mixture over both sides of each cauliflower steak.
4. Place cauliflower steaks on the baking sheet and roast for 20 minutes or until golden brown and tender.
5. Serve the cauliflower steaks with your choice of side vegetables.

Nutrition Information (per serving):

Calories: 120, Protein: 5g, Fat: 7g, Carbohydrates: 12g, Fiber: 6g

Quinoa Stuffed Bell Peppers

Serving: 2

Prep Time: 15 minutes

Cook Time: 30 minutes

Ingredients:

- 2 bell peppers (any color)
- 1/2 cup quinoa, rinsed
- 1 cup low-sodium vegetable broth
- 1 small onion, finely chopped
- 1 garlic clove, minced
- 1/2 cup chopped tomatoes
- 1/4 cup chopped fresh parsley
- Salt and pepper to taste
- 1/4 cup shredded low-fat cheese (optional)

Directions:

1. Set out the oven to 375°F (190°C).

2. Dice the tops off the bell peppers and remove the seeds and membranes. Place them in a baking dish.
3. Place a saucepan, bring the vegetable broth to a boil. Add quinoa, cover, and simmer down for 15 minutes until the compound is absorbed and quinoa is cooked.
4. In a skillet, sauté onion and garlic until softened. Add minced tomatoes and cook for another 2-3 minutes.
5. Combine the cooked quinoa with the sautéed mixture. Stir in chopped parsley, salt, and pepper.
6. Fill up the bell peppers with the quinoa mixture, top with stripped cheese (if using), and cover with the pepper tops.
7. Bake for 25-30 minutes till the peppers are tender.

Calories: 250, Total Fat: 2g, Cholesterol: 0mg, Sodium: 50mg, Total Carbohydrates: 50g, Fiber: 8g, Protein: 8g

Turkey Meatballs with Marinara

Serving: 2

Prep Time: 15 minutes

Cook Time: 25 minutes

Ingredients:

- 8 oz lean ground turkey
- 1/4 cup whole wheat breadcrumbs
- 1 egg
- 1 garlic clove, minced
- 1/4 cup finely chopped onion
- 1 teaspoon Italian seasoning
- Salt and pepper to taste
- 1 cup low-sodium marinara sauce

Directions:

1. Preheat oven to 375°F (190°C).
2. Into a mixing bowl, combine ground turkey, breadcrumbs, egg, minced garlic, chopped onion, Italian seasoning, salt, and pepper. Mix well.
3. Shape the mixture into meatballs (about 1-inch diameter) and place them on a baking sheet layed with parchment paper.
4. Bake for 20-25 minutes till the meatballs are cooked through.
5. Heat the marinara sauce in a saucepan.
6. Serve the turkey meatballs with warm marinara sauce.

Nutrition Information (per serving):

Calories: 280, Total Fat: 12g, Cholesterol: 130mg, Sodium: 550mg, Total Carbohydrates: 15g, Fiber: 3g, Protein: 26g

Baked Cod with Herbs

Serving: 2

Prep Time: 10 minutes

Cook Time: 20 minutes

Ingredients:

- 2 cod fillets (about 6 oz each)
- 2 tablespoons lemon juice
- 1 tablespoon olive oil
- 1 garlic clove, minced
- 1 teaspoon dried parsley
- 1 teaspoon dried thyme
- Salt and pepper to taste
- Lemon wedges for garnish

Directions:

1. Set out the oven to 375°F (190°C).
2. Put the cod fillets in a baking dish.
3. Into a small bowl, mix lemon juice, olive oil, minced garlic, dried

parsley, dried thyme, salt, and pepper.

4. Drizzle the herb mixture over the cod fillets, ensuring they are evenly coated.
5. Bake for 15-20 minutes till the fish flakes easily with a fork.
6. Garnish with lemon wedges before serving.

Calories: 200, Total Fat: 7g, Cholesterol: 70mg, Sodium: 150mg, Total Carbohydrates: 2g, Fiber: 0g, Protein: 30g

Vegetable and Tofu Stir-Fry Noodles

Serving: 2

Prep Time: 20 minutes

Cook Time: 15 minutes

Ingredients:

- 4 oz whole wheat noodles (or soba noodles)
- 1 tablespoon olive oil
- 1 block (14 oz) firm tofu, drained and cubed
- 2 cups mixed vegetables (bell peppers, broccoli, carrots, etc.), sliced
- 2 tablespoons low-sodium soy sauce
- 1 tablespoon rice vinegar
- 1 teaspoon honey or maple syrup
- 1 garlic clove, minced
- 1 teaspoon grated ginger
- Sesame seeds for garnish (optional)

Directions:

1. Cook the noodles according to package instructions. Drain and set aside.
2. Put olive oil in a skillet or wok over medium heat.

3. Lay tofu cubes and stir-fry until golden brown. Reduce the tofu from the skillet and set aside.
4. Into the same skillet, add more oil if needed and stir-fry mixed vegetables until tender-crisp.
5. Take a small bowl, mix soy sauce, rice vinegar, honey (or maple syrup), minced garlic, and grated ginger.
6. Return the tofu to the skillet and add the cooked noodles. Pour the sauce over the compound and toss to combine.
7. Cook for an additional 2-3 minutes until everything is heated through.
8. Grace with sesame seeds if desired before serving.

Calories: 380, Total Fat: 15g, Cholesterol: 0mg, Sodium: 500mg, Total Carbohydrates: 45g, Fiber: 8g, Protein: 20g

Miso-Glazed Tofu

Servings: 2

Prep Time: 10 minutes

Cook Time: 20 minutes

Ingredients:

- 1 block (14 oz) firm tofu, drained and pressed
- 2 tablespoons white miso paste
- 1 tablespoon honey
- 1 tablespoon low-sodium soy sauce
- 1 tablespoon rice vinegar
- 1 teaspoon grated fresh ginger
- 1 clove garlic, minced
- 1 tablespoon sesame oil
- Sesame seeds (for garnish, optional)
- Chopped green onions (for garnish, optional)

Directions:

1. Set out the oven to 400°F (200°C).
2. Cut the tofu into cubes or slices as desired and pat wilt with a paper towel.
3. Into a bowl, whisk together miso paste, honey, soy sauce, rice vinegar, ginger, garlic, and sesame oil.
4. Place tofu in a baking dish lined with parchment paper. Brush the miso mixture over the tofu, ensuring it's coated evenly.
5. Bake for 15-20 minutes or until the tofu is golden and slightly crisp.
6. Season with sesame seeds and chopped green onions if desired. Serve warm.

Calories: 250, Protein: 15g, Fat: 12g, Carbohydrates: 22g, Fiber: 3g

Spaghetti Squash with Marinara

Servings: 2

Prep Time: 10 minutes

Cook Time: 40 minutes

Ingredients:

- 1 medium spaghetti squash
- 2 cups low-fat marinara sauce
- 1 tablespoon olive oil
- Salt and pepper to taste
- Fresh basil leaves (for garnish, optional)
- Grated Parmesan cheese (optional)

Directions:

1. Set out the oven to 400°F (200°C).
2. Dice the spaghetti squash in half lengthwise and scoop out the seeds. Dribble olive oil and sprinkle with salt and pepper.
3. Lay the squash halves cut side down on a baking sheet lined with parchment paper. Roast for 30-40 minutes until tender.
4. Once it's made, use a fork to scrape the flesh of the squash into strands.
5. Put the marinara sauce in a saucepan over medium heat. Add the spaghetti squash strands and toss to coat.
6. Set out hot, garnished with fresh basil leaves and grated Parmesan cheese if desired.

Calories: 180, Protein: 4g, Fat: 6g, Carbohydrates: 28g, Fiber: 7g

Chickpea and Vegetable Curry

Servings: 2

Prep Time: 10 minutes

Cook Time: 25 minutes

Ingredients:

- 1 can (15 oz) chickpeas, drained off and rinsed
- 1 cup diced mixed vegetables (bell peppers, carrots, broccoli, etc.)
- 1 small onion, finely chopped
- 2 cloves garlic, minced
- 1 teaspoon grated fresh ginger
- 1 tablespoon curry powder
- 1 can (14 oz) low-fat coconut milk
- 1 tablespoon olive oil
- Salt and pepper to taste
- Fresh cilantro (for garnish, optional)
- Cooked rice (for serving, optional)

Directions:

1. Lay the olive oil in a pan over medium heat. Add chopped onions, garlic, and ginger. Sauté until fragrant.
2. Add mixed vegetables and chickpeas, stirring occasionally for 3-4 minutes.

3. Sprinkle curry powder over the mixture and stir well.
4. Lay in the coconut milk, bring to a simmer, and stir it for about 15 minutes until vegetables are edible and the sauce has thickened slightly.
5. Season with salt and pepper to taste.
6. Serve hot over rice if desired, garnished with fresh cilantro.

Calories: 320, Protein: 12g, Fat: 15g, Carbohydrates: 35g, Fiber: 9g

4. Stuff each zucchini boat with the quinoa mixture.
5. Place the boats on a baking sheet lined with parchment paper. Bake for 20 minutes.
6. Remove from the oven, sprinkle shredded mozzarella on top, and bake for an additional 5 minutes until cheese melts.
7. Garnish with chopped parsley before serving.

Calories: 220, Protein: 14g, Fat: 8g, Carbohydrates: 24g, Fiber: 6g

Zucchini Boats

Servings: 2

Prep Time: 15 minutes

Cook Time: 25 minutes

Ingredients:

- 2 medium zucchinis
- ½ cup cooked quinoa
- ½ cup diced tomatoes
- ½ cup cooked lean ground turkey (optional)
- ¼ cup low-fat shredded mozzarella cheese
- 1 tablespoon olive oil
- 1 teaspoon Italian seasoning
- Salt and pepper to taste
- Chopped parsley (for garnish, optional)

Directions:

1. Set off the oven to 375°F (190°C).
2. Cut the zucchinis in half lengthwise and scoop out the centers to create a hollow "boat."
3. In a bowl, mix together quinoa, diced tomatoes, cooked ground turkey (if using), olive oil, Italian seasoning, salt, and pepper.

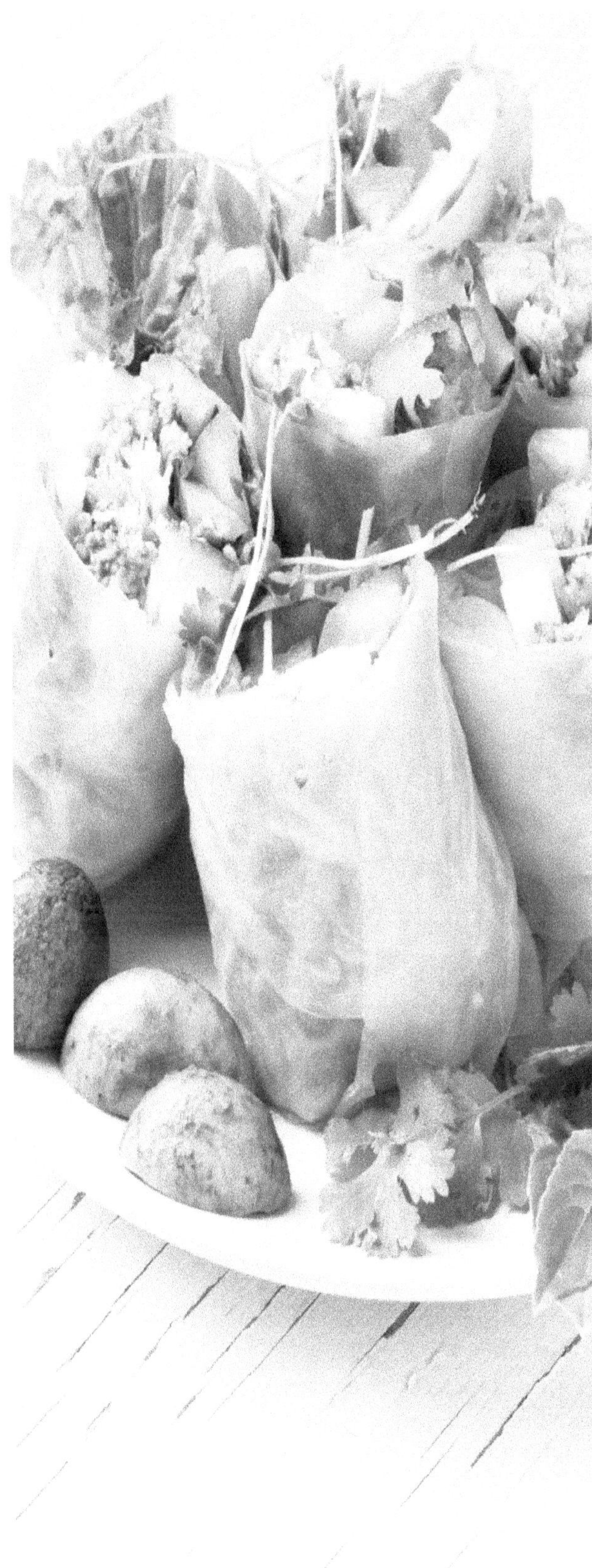

Savory

Vegetable Soup

Serving: 2

Prep Time: 10 minutes

Cook Time: 25 minutes

Ingredients:

- 1 tablespoon olive oil
- 1 onion, chopped
- 2 carrots, diced
- 2 celery stalks, sliced
- 2 cups low-sodium vegetable broth
- 1 cup diced tomatoes (canned or fresh)
- 1 cup chopped spinach or kale
- Salt and pepper to taste

Directions:

1. Sprinkle olive oil in a pot over medium heat. Add chopped onion, carrots, and celery. Sauté for 5-7 minutes until slightly softened.
2. Gush in the vegetable broth and diced tomatoes. Bring to a simmer down and cook for 15 minutes.
3. Add chopped spinach or kale. Simmer for an additional 5 minutes.
4. Season with salt and pepper to taste. Serve warm.

Nutrition Information (per serving):

Calories: 120, Total Fat: 5g, Sodium: 320mg, Carbohydrates: 18g, Fiber: 5g, Protein: 4g

Stuffed Bell Peppers

Serving: 2

Prep Time: 15 minutes

Cook Time: 30 minutes

Ingredients:

- 2 bell peppers (preferred color), halved and seeded
- 1 cup cooked quinoa
- ½ cup cooked lean ground turkey or chicken
- ½ cup chopped zucchini
- ½ cup chopped tomatoes
- 2 tablespoons chopped fresh parsley
- 1 teaspoon olive oil
- Salt and pepper to taste

Directions:

1. Preset the oven to 375°F (190°C).
2. In a bowl, mix together cooked quinoa, ground turkey or chicken, chopped zucchini, tomatoes, parsley, olive oil, salt, and pepper.
3. Load up each bell pepper half with the mixture.
4. Lay the stuffed peppers on a baking sheet and bake for 25-30 minutes till the peppers are tender.

Nutrition Information (per serving):

Calories: 250, Total Fat: 8g, Sodium: 180mg, Carbohydrates: 30g, Fiber: 8g, Protein: 18g

Mushroom Risotto

Serving: 2

Prep Time: 10 minutes

Cook Time: 30 minutes

Ingredients:

- 1 cup Arborio rice
- 2 cups low-sodium chicken or vegetable broth
- 1 tablespoon olive oil
- 1 cup sliced mushrooms
- 1 small onion, finely chopped
- 2 cloves garlic, minced
- ¼ cup grated Parmesan cheese (optional)
- Salt and pepper to taste

Directions:

1. Into a saucepan, heat the chicken or vegetable broth and store it warm on low heat.
2. Take a separate pan, heat olive oil over medium heat. Add carved onion and saute until translucent, about 3 minutes. Add minced garlic and sliced mushrooms, cook for 5 minutes.
3. Place Arborio rice to the pan and stir for 2 minutes until it's coated with the oil and slightly toasted.
4. Gradually add the warm broth, ½ cup at a time, stirring frequently until absorbed before adding more. Keep up until the rice is tender and creamy (about 20-25 minutes).
5. Stir in grated Parmesan cheese (if using), salt, and pepper. Serve warm.

Nutrition Information (per serving):

Calories: 350, Total Fat: 7g, Sodium: 480mg, Carbohydrates: 60g, Fiber: 3g, Protein: 9g

Zucchini and Carrot Fritters

Serving: 2

Prep Time: 15 minutes

Cook Time: 15 minutes

Ingredients:

- 1 zucchini, grated
- 1 carrot, grated
- 1 egg
- 2 tablespoons wheat flour or almond flour
- 1 tablespoon olive oil
- Salt and pepper to taste

Directions:

1. Place grated zucchini and carrot in a clean kitchen towel and squeeze out excess moisture.
2. In a bowl, mix together grated vegetables, egg, and flour. Season with salt and pepper.
3. Add up olive oil in a skillet over medium heat.
4. Spoon the mixture onto the skillet, flattening to form fritters. Cook for 3-4 minutes per side until golden brown.
5. Reduce from the skillet and place on a paper towel to drain excess oil. Serve warm.

Nutrition Information (per serving):

Calories: 180, Total Fat: 10g, Sodium: 120mg, Carbohydrates: 18g, Fiber: 4g, Protein: 6g

Spinach and Feta Stuffed Mushrooms

Serving: 2-3

Prep Time: 15 minutes

Cook Time: 20 minutes

Ingredients:

- 10-12 large mushrooms
- 1 cup fresh spinach, chopped
- 1/2 cup crumbled feta cheese
- 2 cloves garlic, minced
- 2 tablespoons olive oil
- Salt and pepper to taste

Directions:

1. Preheat oven to 350°F (175°C). Clean mushrooms and remove stems, creating a hollow center.
2. Into a skillet, heat olive oil over medium heat. Add garlic and sauté for 1-2 minutes.
3. Add carved spinach to the skillet and cook until wilted, around 2-3 minutes. Remove from heat.
4. In a bowl, mix together the sautéed spinach, feta cheese, salt, and pepper.
5. Spoon the mixture into the hollowed-out mushrooms.
6. Lay the stuffed mushrooms on a baking sheet and bake for 15-20 minutes till mushrooms are soft.

Nutrition Information (per serving):

Calories: 120, Total Fat: 8g, Cholesterol: 15mg, Sodium: 180mg, Total Carbohydrates: 6g, Protein: 6g

Cucumber Dill Salad

Serving: 2-3

Prep Time: 10 minutes

No Cook Time

Ingredients:

- 2 medium cucumbers, thinly sliced
- 1/4 cup plain Greek yogurt
- 1 tablespoon fresh dill, chopped
- 1 tablespoon lemon juice
- Salt and pepper to taste

Directions:

1. In a bowl, combine sliced cucumbers, Greek yogurt, fresh dill, lemon juice, salt, and pepper.
2. Toss gently until cucumbers are evenly coated with the dressing.
3. Cool it in the refrigerator for 15-20 minutes before serving.

Nutrition Information (per serving):

Calories: 40, Total Fat: 0.5g, Cholesterol: 0mg, Sodium: 20mg, Total Carbohydrates: 7g, Protein: 3g

Ratatouille

Serving: 3-4

Prep Time: 15 minutes

Cook Time: 30 minutes

Ingredients:

- 1 small eggplant, diced
- 1 zucchini, diced
- 1 yellow squash, diced
- 1 bell pepper, diced
- 1 onion, diced
- 2 cloves garlic, minced
- 2 tablespoons olive oil
- 1 can (14 oz) diced tomatoes
- 1 teaspoon dried basil
- 1 teaspoon dried oregano
- Salt and pepper to taste

Directions:

1. Into a large skillet, heat up olive oil over medium heat. Add onion and garlic, sauté until translucent.
2. Add diced eggplant, zucchini, yellow squash, and bell pepper to the skillet. Cook for 5-7 minutes until slightly tender.
3. Stir in diced tomatoes, dried basil, dried oregano, salt, and pepper. Simmer down for 15-20 minutes until vegetables are cooked but not mushy.

Nutrition Information (per serving):

Calories: 120, Total Fat: 6g, Cholesterol: 0mg, Sodium: 220mg, Total Carbohydrates: 18g, Protein: 3g

Cauliflower Mash

Serving: 2-3

Prep Time: 10 minutes

Cook Time: 15 minutes

Ingredients:

- 1 head cauliflower, cut into florets
- 2 cloves garlic, minced
- 2 tablespoons unsalted butter
- Salt and pepper to taste
- 2 tablespoons chopped chives (optional)

Directions:

1. Steam or boil cauliflower florets and garlic until very tender, about 10-12 minutes.
2. Drain excess water and transfer cauliflower and garlic to a bowl.
3. Add butter, salt, and pepper. Mush with a potato masher or blend until smooth.
4. Sprinkle chopped chives on top if desired before serving.

Nutrition Information (per serving):

Calories: 70, Total Fat: 4g, Cholesterol: 10mg, Sodium: 40mg, Total Carbohydrates: 8g, Protein: 3g

Vegetable Kebabs

Servings: 2

Prep Time: 15 minutes

Cook Time: 10 minutes

Ingredients:

- 1 bell pepper, diced into chunks
- 1 zucchini, sliced
- 1 onion, diced into chunks
- 8 cherry tomatoes
- 8 button mushrooms
- 2 tablespoons olive oil
- Salt and pepper to taste

Directions:

1. Preset the grill or oven to medium-high heat.
2. Thread the vegetables onto skewers, alternating between them.

3. Wash the kebabs with olive oil and season with salt and pepper.
4. Grill or bake for about 10 minutes, turning at times until the vegetables are tender and slightly charred.
5. Serve warm.

Calories: 180, Fat: 10g, Carbohydrates: 20g, Fiber: 6g, Protein: 4g

Broccoli and Cheddar Soup

Servings: 2

Prep Time: 10 minutes

Cook Time: 20 minutes

Ingredients:

- 2 cups chopped broccoli florets
- 1 small onion, chopped
- 2 cloves garlic, minced
- 2 cups low-sodium chicken or vegetable broth
- 1 cup low-fat cheddar cheese, grated
- Salt and pepper to taste

Directions:

1. In a pot, sauté the onion and garlic until softened.
2. Add the broccoli and broth, then bring to a boil. Reduce heat and simmer down for about 10-15 minutes until broccoli is tender.
3. Use an immersion blender or transfer to a grinder to puree the soup until smooth.
4. Ladle in the grated cheddar cheese until melted and smooth.
5. Season with salt and pepper to taste.
6. Serve hot.

Nutrition Information: (per serving)

Calories: 220, Fat: 10g, Carbohydrates: 15g, Fiber: 5g, Protein: 15g

Sweet Potato Rounds

Servings: 2

Prep Time: 10 minutes

Cook Time: 20 minutes

Ingredients:

- 2 medium sweet potatoes, sliced into rounds
- 2 tablespoons olive oil
- 1 teaspoon paprika
- 1 teaspoon garlic powder
- Salt and pepper to taste

Directions:

1. Preset oven to 400°F (200°C) and line a baking sheet with parchment paper.
2. Into a bowl, toss the sweet potato rounds with olive oil, paprika, garlic powder, salt, and pepper until evenly coated.
3. Put the rounds on the baking sheet in a single layer.
4. Cook slowly for 20 minutes or until the sweet potatoes are tender and slightly crispy.
5. Serve warm.

Nutrition Information: (per serving)

Calories: 200, Fat: 7g, Carbohydrates: 35g, Fiber: 6g, Protein: 3g

Greek Yogurt Dip with Veggies

Servings: 4

Prep Time: 10 minutes

Ingredients:

- 1 cup plain Greek yogurt
- 1 tablespoon lemon juice
- 1 clove garlic, minced

- 1 teaspoon dried dill
- Salt and pepper to taste
- Assorted chopped vegetables for dipping (carrots, cucumber, bell peppers, etc.)

Directions:

1. Take a bowl, mix together the Greek yogurt, lemon juice, minced garlic, dried dill, salt, and pepper until well combined.
2. Adjust seasoning to taste.
3. Serve the dip with assorted chopped vegetables.

Nutrition Information: (per serving, dip only)

Calories: 35, Fat: 0g, Carbohydrates: 3g, Fiber: 0g, Protein: 6g

Cabbage Rolls

Servings: 2-3

Prep Time: 20 minutes

Cook Time: 40 minutes

Ingredients:

- 6 large cabbage leaves
- 1 cup lean ground turkey or chicken
- 1/2 cup cooked white rice
- 1/4 cup finely chopped onion
- 1/4 cup low-sodium chicken broth
- 1 teaspoon olive oil
- 1/2 teaspoon dried thyme
- Salt and pepper to taste
- 1 cup low-fat tomato sauce (optional)

Directions:

1. Preheat oven to 350°F (175°C).
2. Take a skillet over medium heat, add olive oil and sauté onions until translucent.
3. Add ground turkey or chicken to the skillet and cook until browned.
4. Stir in cooked rice, dried thyme, salt, and pepper. Mix well.
5. Place cabbage leaves in boiling water for 2-3 minutes until softened. Remove and drain.
6. Take each cabbage leaf and fill with the meat mixture, rolling them tightly.
7. Place the rolls seam side down in a baking dish. Pour chicken broth over the rolls.
8. Wrap the dish with foil and bake for 25-30 minutes.
9. Optionally, spoon tomato sauce over the cabbage rolls and bake uncovered for an extra 10 minutes.
10. Serve warm.

Nutrition Information (per serving):

Calories: 220, Protein: 18g, Carbohydrates: 17g, Fat: 8g, Fiber: 4g

Stuffed Tomatoes

Servings: 2

Prep Time: 15 minutes

Cook Time: 25 minutes

Ingredients:

- 2 large tomatoes
- 1/2 cup cooked quinoa
- 1/4 cup chopped bell peppers
- 1/4 cup chopped cucumber
- 2 tablespoons chopped fresh parsley
- 1 tablespoon olive oil
- 1 tablespoon lemon juice
- Salt and pepper to taste

Directions:

1. Preheat oven to 375°F (190°C).
2. Carve the tops off the tomatoes and carefully scoop out the pulp, leaving a shell.

3. Take a bowl, mix together quinoa, bell peppers, cucumber, parsley, olive oil, lemon juice, salt, and pepper.
4. Stuff each tomato with the quinoa compound.
5. Place the packed tomatoes in a baking dish and bake for 20-25 minutes until tomatoes are tender.
6. Serve warm.

Nutrition Information (per serving):

Calories: 180, Protein: 5g, Carbohydrates: 25g, Fat: 7g, Fiber: 5g

Roasted Brussels Sprouts

Servings: 2

Prep Time: 10 minutes

Cook Time: 25 minutes

Ingredients:

- 2 cups Brussels sprouts, trimmed and halved
- 2 tablespoons olive oil
- 2 cloves garlic, minced
- 1/2 teaspoon paprika
- Salt and pepper to taste

Directions:

1. Preheat oven to 400°F (200°C).
2. Take a bowl, toss Brussels sprouts with olive oil, minced garlic, paprika, salt, and pepper until coated.
3. Roll out the Brussels sprouts on a baking sheet in a single layer.
4. Cook in the oven for 20-25 minutes, stirring halfway through, until sprouts are tender and slightly browned.
5. Serve hot.

Nutrition Information (per serving):

Calories: 150, Protein: 5g, Carbohydrates: 12g, Fat: 10g, Fiber: 5g

Eggplant Chips

Servings: 2

Prep Time: 15 minutes

Cook Time: 20 minutes

Ingredients:

- 1 medium eggplant, thinly sliced
- 2 tablespoons olive oil
- 1/4 teaspoon garlic powder
- 1/4 teaspoon smoked paprika
- Salt and pepper to taste

Directions:

1. Preheat oven to 375°F (190°C).
2. Place eggplant carves on paper towels and sprinkle with salt. Let sit for 10 minutes to draw out excess moisture.
3. Pat the eggplant slices dry and place them in a bowl.
4. Dribble olive oil over the slices and sprinkle with garlic powder, charred paprika, salt, and pepper. Toss to coat evenly.
5. Arrange the carvings on a baking sheet in a single layer.
6. Bake for 15-20 minutes, rolling over halfway through, until the eggplant is friable and golden brown.
7. Reduce from oven and let cool slightly before serving.

Nutrition Information (per serving):

Calories: 120, Protein: 2g, Carbohydrates: 8g, Fat: 9g, Fiber: 4g

Cucumber Avocado Rolls

Servings: 2

Prep Time: 15 minutes

Ingredients:

- 1 large cucumber
- 1 ripe avocado

- 1 small red bell pepper, thinly sliced
- 1 carrot, julienned
- 2 tablespoons fresh cilantro, chopped
- Juice of 1 lime
- Salt and pepper to taste

Directions:

1. Skin off the cucumber and slice it lengthwise into thin strips using a vegetable peeler.
2. Take a bowl, mash the avocado with lime juice, salt, and pepper.
3. Roll out a thin layer of mashed avocado onto each cucumber strip.
4. Place a few slices of bell pepper, julienned carrots, and chopped cilantro on top.
5. Roll up the cucumber strips and secure them with a toothpick.
6. Serve immediately and enjoy!

Nutrition Information (per serving):

Calories: 150, Total Fat: 10g, Carbohydrates: 15g, Fiber: 8g, Protein: 3g

Cauliflower Buffalo Bites

Servings: 2

Prep Time: 10 minutes

Cook Time: 20 minutes

Ingredients:

- 1 small curd of cauliflower, cut into florets
- 1/2 cup almond flour
- 1 teaspoon garlic powder
- 1 teaspoon paprika
- Salt and pepper to taste
- 1/4 cup hot sauce
- 2 tablespoons olive oil

Directions:

1. Preheat oven to 450°F (230°C). Line a baking sheet with parchment paper.
2. Take a bowl, mix almond flour, garlic powder, paprika, salt, and pepper.
3. Toss cauliflower florets in olive oil, then coat them with the almond flour mixture.
4. Rest the coated florets on the baking paper and bake for 15-20 minutes or until crispy.
5. In a separate bowl, mix hot sauce with a little olive oil.
6. Once the cauliflower is done, toss it in the hot sauce mixture until well coated.
7. Serve warm and enjoy these guilt-free buffalo bites!

Nutrition Information (per serving):

Calories: 180, Total Fat: 12g, Carbohydrates: 12g, Fiber: 6g, Protein: 7g

Greek Orzo Salad

Servings: 2

Prep Time: 15 minutes

Cook Time: 10 minutes

Ingredients:

- 1 cup cooked orzo pasta
- 1 cucumber, diced
- 1 cup cherry tomatoes, halved
- 1/2 red onion, finely chopped
- 1/4 cup Kalamata olives, sliced
- 2 tablespoons fresh parsley, chopped
- 2 tablespoons olive oil
- 1 tablespoon red wine vinegar
- Salt and pepper to taste

Directions:

1. In a large bowl, combine cooked orzo, diced cucumber, cherry

tomatoes, red onion, olives, and parsley.

2. In a small bowl, whip olive oil, red wine vinegar, salt, & bell pepper to make the seasoning.
3. Gush the dressing over the salad and toss gently to coat.
4. Serve chilled or at room temperature. Enjoy this refreshing Greek orzo salad!

Calories: 280, Total Fat: 14g, Carbohydrates: 34g, Fiber: 5g, Protein: 6g

Artichoke and Spinach Dip

Servings: 4

Prep Time: 10 minutes

Cook Time: 20 minutes

Ingredients:

- 1 can (14 oz) artichoke hearts, drained off and chopped
- 1 cup frozen carved spinach, thawed and drained
- 1/2 cup plain Greek yogurt
- 1/4 cup grated Parmesan cheese
- 1/4 cup low-fat mayonnaise
- 1 clove garlic, minced
- Salt and pepper to taste

Directions:

1. Preheat oven to 375°F (190°C).
2. Take a mixing bowl, combine chopped artichoke hearts, spinach, Greek yogurt, Parmesan cheese, mayonnaise, minced garlic, salt, and pepper.
3. Remove the mixture to an oven-safe dish and spread it evenly.
4. Bake for 20 minutes up until the top is golden and bubbly.
5. Serve warm with whole grain crackers or sliced vegetables.

Nutrition Information (per serving):

Calories: 150, Total Fat: 8g, Carbohydrates: 10g, Fiber: 4g, Protein: 8g

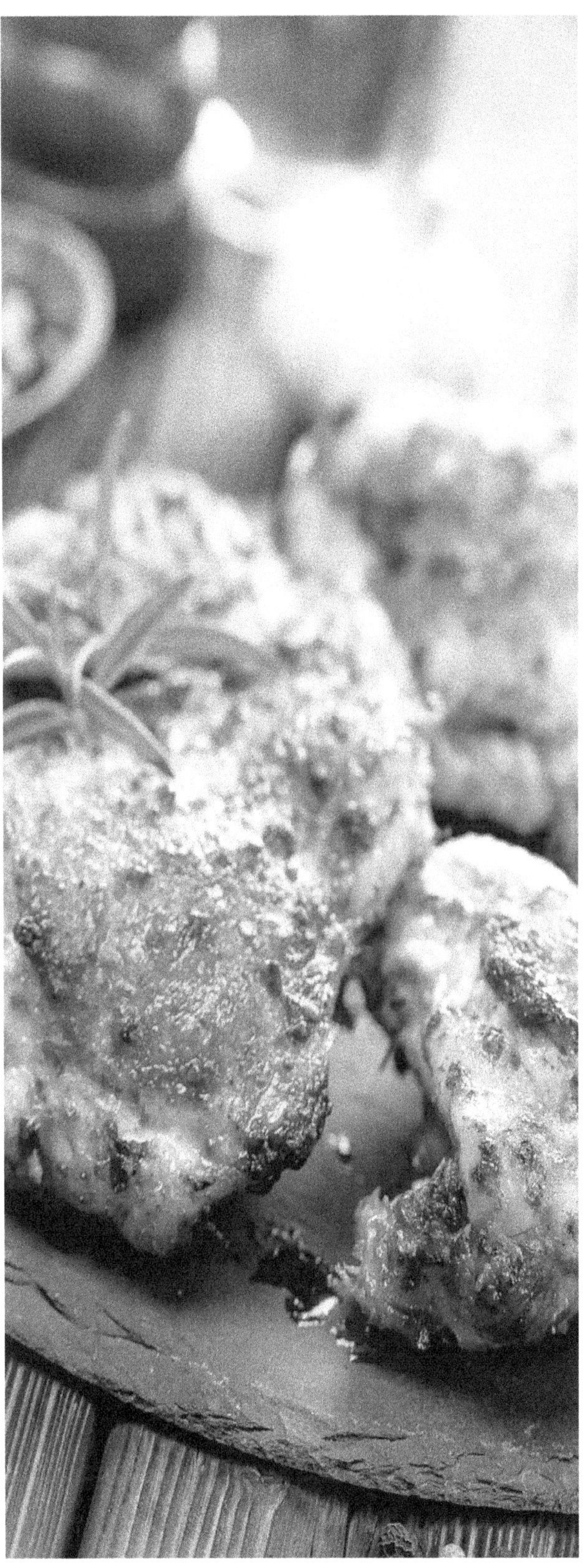

Poultry

Baked Lemon Herb Chicken Breast

Servings: 2

Prep Time: 10 minutes

Cook Time: 25 minutes

Ingredients:

- 2 boneless, skinless chicken breasts
- 2 tablespoons olive oil
- 1 lemon (juice and zest)
- 2 cloves garlic, minced
- 1 teaspoon dried thyme
- 1 teaspoon dried rosemary
- Salt and pepper to taste

Directions:

1. Place the oven to 375°F (190°C).
2. Into a bowl, mix olive oil, lemon zest, lemon juice, minced garlic, thyme, rosemary, salt, and pepper.
3. Settle the chicken breasts in a baking dish and pour the lemon herb mixture over them, ensuring they are evenly coated.
4. Bake in the preset oven for about 25 minutes or until the chicken is cooked through (reaches an inward temperature of 165°F or 74°C).
5. Remove from the oven, let it rest for a few minutes, then serve with a side of steamed vegetables or rice.

Nutrition Information (per serving):

Calories: 250, Protein: 30g, Carbohydrates: 2g, Fat: 13g, Fiber: 1g

Turkey and Vegetable Skewers

Servings: 2

Prep Time: 15 minutes

Cook Time: 10 minutes

Ingredients:

- 1 turkey breast, cut into chunks
- 1 zucchini, sliced
- 1 bell pepper, cut into squares
- 8 cherry tomatoes
- 2 tablespoons olive oil
- 1 teaspoon paprika
- 1 teaspoon garlic powder
- Salt and pepper to taste

Directions:

1. Preheat the grill or broiler.
2. In a bowl, mix olive oil, paprika, garlic powder, salt, and pepper.
3. Thread the turkey chunks, zucchini slices, bell pepper, and cherry tomatoes onto skewers.
4. Sweep the skewers with the olive oil mixture.
5. Broil the skewers for about 10 minutes, turning occasionally, until the turkey is cooked through and vegetables are tender.
6. Serve the skewers with a side salad or quinoa.

Nutrition Information (per serving):

Calories: 280, Protein: 32g, Carbohydrates: 7g, Fat: 13g, Fiber: 2g

Chicken and Vegetable Stir-Fry

Servings: 2

Prep Time: 15 minutes

Cook Time: 15 minutes

Ingredients:

- 2 boneless, skinless chicken breasts, sliced
- 1 cup broccoli florets
- 1 bell pepper, sliced
- 1 carrot, sliced
- 2 tablespoons low-sodium soy sauce
- 1 tablespoon honey

- 1 tablespoon olive oil
- 2 cloves garlic, minced
- 1 teaspoon ginger, grated
- Salt and pepper to taste

1. Put olive oil in a pan or wok over medium-high heat.
2. Place the chicken slices and cook until lightly browned.
3. Add minced garlic, grated ginger, broccoli, bell pepper, and carrot to the pan. Stir-fry for a few minutes until vegetables are tender-crisp.
4. Take a small bowl, mix soy sauce and honey. Pour this mixture over the stir-fry and toss to coat evenly.
5. Cook for an additional 2-3 minutes until everything is heated through and well combined.
6. Season with salt and pepper to taste.
7. Serve hot with brown rice or quinoa.

Nutrition Information (per serving):

Calories: 290, Protein: 30g, Carbohydrates: 16g, Fat: 11g, Fiber: 4g

Herb-Roasted Turkey Tenderloin

Servings: 2

Prep Time: 10 minutes

Cook Time: 30 minutes

Ingredients:

- 1 turkey tenderloin
- 2 tablespoons olive oil
- 1 teaspoon dried thyme
- 1 teaspoon dried oregano
- 1 teaspoon dried sage
- Salt and pepper to taste

Directions:

1. Place the oven to 400°F (200°C).
2. Wash the turkey tenderloin with olive oil and season with thyme, oregano, sage, salt, and pepper.
3. Place the seasoned turkey in a baking dish.
4. Roast in the preset oven for about 30 minutes or until the turkey reaches an inward temperature of 165°F (74°C).
5. Remove from the oven, let it lay for a few minutes, then slice and serve with steamed vegetables or a side salad.

Nutrition Information (per serving):

Calories: 240, Protein: 30g, Carbohydrates: 0g, Fat: 13g, Fiber: 0g

Chicken Lettuce Wraps

Servings: 2

Prep Time: 15 minutes

Cook Time: 15 minutes

Ingredients:

- 1 tablespoon olive oil
- 1 pound ground chicken
- 1/2 cup diced bell peppers
- 1/4 cup diced water chestnuts
- 2 tablespoons low-sodium soy sauce
- 1 tablespoon rice vinegar
- 1 tablespoon honey
- 1 teaspoon minced ginger
- 1 teaspoon minced garlic
- Salt and pepper to taste
- 1 head iceberg or butter lettuce, leaves parted

Directions:

1. Spout olive oil in a skillet over medium heat. Add chopped up chicken and cook until no longer pink.
2. Stir in bell peppers, water chestnuts, soy sauce, rice vinegar, honey,

ginger, garlic, salt, and pepper. Cook for 5-7 minutes up until vegetables are tender and flavors combine.

3. Spoon the chicken mixture into individual lettuce leaves, creating wraps.
4. Serve immediately and enjoy.

Nutrition Information (per serving):

Calories: 320, Protein: 25g, Carbohydrates: 12g, Fat: 18g, Fiber: 3g

Grilled Citrus Chicken Thighs

Servings: 2

Prep Time: 10 minutes

Cook Time: 15 minutes

Ingredients:

- 2 boneless, skinless chicken thighs
- Zest and juice of 1 lemon
- Zest and juice of 1 orange
- 1 tablespoon olive oil
- 1 teaspoon honey
- 1 teaspoon minced garlic
- Salt and pepper to taste

Directions:

1. In a bowl, mix lemon zest, orange zest, lemon juice, orange juice, olive oil, honey, garlic, salt, and pepper.
2. Drench the chicken thighs in this mixture for at least 30 minutes in the refrigerator.
3. Preheat the grill to medium-high heat. Grill chicken thighs for about 6-8 minutes per side or until cooked through.
4. Remove from the grill, let rest for a few minutes, then serve.

Nutrition Information (per serving):

Calories: 280, Protein: 28g, Carbohydrates: 8g, Fat: 14g, Fiber: 1g

Turkey and Spinach Meatballs

Servings: 2

Prep Time: 20 minutes

Cook Time: 20 minutes

Ingredients:

- 1/2 pound ground turkey
- 1 cup chopped spinach
- 1/4 cup breadcrumbs (use gluten-free if needed)
- 1 egg
- 1 tablespoon chopped fresh parsley
- 1 teaspoon minced garlic
- 1/2 teaspoon dried oregano
- Salt and pepper to taste
- 1 tablespoon olive oil

Directions:

1. Preset the oven to 375°F (190°C). Line a baking sheet with parchment paper.
2. In a bowl, combine ground turkey, chopped spinach, breadcrumbs, egg, parsley, garlic, oregano, salt, and pepper. Mix until well combined.
3. Shape the mixture into meatballs and place them on the prepared baking sheet.
4. Dribble olive oil over the meatballs and bake for 15-20 minutes until they are cooked through and golden brown.
5. Serve with a side of cooked vegetables or rice, if desired.

Nutrition Information (per serving):

Calories: 280, Protein: 25g, Carbohydrates: 10g, Fat: 15g, Fiber: 2g

Servings: 2

Prep Time: 10 minutes

Cook Time: 35 minutes

Ingredients:

- 4 chicken drumsticks
- 2 tablespoons olive oil
- 1 tablespoon chopped fresh rosemary
- 1 teaspoon minced garlic
- Salt and pepper to taste

Directions:

1. Preset the oven to 400°F (200°C). Line a baking dish with parchment paper.
2. In a bowl, mix together olive oil, chopped rosemary, minced garlic, salt, and pepper.
3. Coat chicken drumsticks evenly with the mixture.
4. Place the drumsticks in the baking dish and bake for about 30-35 minutes or until the chicken is golden brown and cooked through.
5. Serve hot with your choice of steamed vegetables or a side salad.

Nutrition Information (per serving):

Calories: 320, Protein: 24g, Carbohydrates: 0g, Fat: 24g, Fiber: 0g

Chicken and Rice Soup

Servings: 2

Prep Time: 10 minutes

Cook Time: 30 minutes

Ingredients:

- 1 boneless, skinless chicken breast, diced
- 1 cup cooked white rice
- 4 cups low-sodium chicken broth
- 1 carrot, diced
- 1 celery stalk, diced
- 1/2 onion, finely chopped
- 1 teaspoon dried parsley
- Salt and pepper to taste

Directions:

1. Into a pot, bring chicken broth to a simmer over medium heat.
2. Add diced chicken, carrot, celery, onion, and dried parsley to the simmering broth.
3. Roast it for 20-25 minutes until chicken is cooked through and vegetables are tender.
4. Stir in cooked white rice and let it simmer for an additional 5 minutes.
5. Season with salt and pepper to taste.
6. Serve warm.

Nutrition Information (per serving):

Calories: 250, Protein: 20g, Carbohydrates: 25g, Fat: 6g

Turkey and Quinoa Stuffed Peppers

Servings: 2

Prep Time: 15 minutes

Cook Time: 40 minutes

Ingredients:

- 2 large bell peppers, halved and seeds removed
- 1/2 cup cooked quinoa
- 1/2 pound ground turkey
- 1/2 cup diced tomatoes
- 1/4 cup chopped fresh parsley
- 1 teaspoon garlic powder
- Salt and pepper to taste
- 1/4 cup low-sodium chicken broth

Directions:

1. Preheat oven to 375°F (190°C).

2. In a bowl, mix together cooked quinoa, ground turkey, diced tomatoes, chopped parsley, garlic powder, salt, and pepper.
3. Fill each bell pepper half with the turkey-quinoa mixture.
4. Put down the stuffed peppers in a baking dish and gush chicken broth into the bottom of the dish.
5. Wrap the dish with foil and bake for 30-35 minutes until peppers are tender and filling is cooked through.
6. Serve hot.

Nutrition Information (per serving):

Calories: 320, Protein: 25g, Carbohydrates: 25g, Fat: 12g

Grilled Lemon Herb Turkey Burgers

Servings: 2

Prep Time: 10 minutes

Cook Time: 15 minutes

Ingredients:

- 1/2 pound ground turkey
- 1 tablespoon chopped fresh parsley
- 1 teaspoon lemon zest
- 1 teaspoon dried oregano
- Salt and pepper to taste
- Lettuce leaves, tomato slices (optional for serving)

Directions:

1. Preheat grill or stovetop grill pan over medium heat.
2. In a bowl, mix together ground turkey, chopped parsley, lemon zest, dried oregano, salt, and pepper.
3. Carve up the mixture into two portions and shape into burger patties.
4. Grill the turkey burgers for about 6-7 minutes per side, or until cooked through.
5. Serve on lettuce leaves with optional tomato slices.

Nutrition Information (per serving):

Calories: 200, Protein: 30g, Carbohydrates: 2g, Fat: 8g

Chicken and Veggie Lettuce Wraps

Servings: 2

Prep Time: 15 minutes

Cook Time: 10 minutes

Ingredients:

- 1 boneless, skinless chicken breast, diced
- 1 tablespoon olive oil
- 1/2 onion, finely chopped
- 1 garlic clove, minced
- 1 cup mixed vegetables (bell peppers, carrots, mushrooms), diced
- 2 tablespoons low-sodium soy sauce
- 1 teaspoon honey
- Lettuce leaves for wrapping

Directions:

1. Put in olive oil in a skillet over medium heat.
2. Add carved chicken and cook until no longer pink, then remove from the skillet and set aside.
3. In the same skillet, sauté onion and garlic until fragrant.
4. Put in the mixed vegetables and cook for 3-4 minutes until tender.
5. Return the cooked chicken to the skillet.
6. Stir in low-sodium soy sauce and honey, cooking for an additional 2 minutes.

7. Spoon the chicken and vegetable mixture onto lettuce leaves and wrap.

Calories: 220, Protein: 25g, Carbohydrates: 10g, Fat: 8g

Turkey and Vegetable Chili

Servings: 2

Prep Time: 15 minutes

Cook Time: 30 minutes

Ingredients:

- 1 tablespoon olive oil
- 1/2 pound ground turkey
- 1/2 cup diced onion
- 1/2 cup diced bell pepper
- 1 can (14 oz) low-sodium diced tomatoes
- 1 can (14 oz) low-sodium kidney beans, drained and rinsed
- 1 teaspoon chili powder
- 1/2 teaspoon cumin
- Salt and pepper to taste

Directions:

1. Put in olive oil in a skillet over medium heat. Add ground turkey and cook until browned.
2. Add diced onion and bell pepper. Cook until vegetables are tender.
3. Stir in diced tomatoes, kidney beans, chili powder, cumin, salt, and pepper.
4. Simmer for 20-25 minutes, stirring occasionally.
5. Serve warm.

Nutrition Information (per serving):

Calories: 320, Protein: 25g, Fat: 12g, Carbohydrates: 28g, Fiber: 9g

Oven-Baked Panko-Crusted Chicken Tenders

Servings: 2

Prep Time: 10 minutes

Cook Time: 20 minutes

Ingredients:

- 2 boneless, skinned chicken breasts, cut into strips
- 1/2 cup whole wheat panko breadcrumbs
- 1 teaspoon garlic powder
- 1/2 teaspoon paprika
- Salt and pepper to taste
- Cooking spray

Directions:

1. Preheat oven to 400°F (200°C). Fix a baking sheet with parchment paper and lightly coat with cooking spray.
2. In a shallow bowl, mix panko breadcrumbs, garlic powder, paprika, salt, and pepper.
3. Coat each chicken strip in the breadcrumb mixture and place on the prepared baking sheet.
4. Bake for 18-20 minutes or till chicken is cooked through and crispy.
5. Serve warm with a side of non-fat yogurt or applesauce for dipping.

Nutrition Information (per serving):

Calories: 250, Protein: 30g, Fat: 4g, Carbohydrates: 21g, Fiber: 3g

Lemon Garlic Turkey Cutlets

Servings: 2

Prep Time: 10 minutes

Cook Time: 15 minutes

Ingredients:

- 2 turkey cutlets
- 2 tablespoons olive oil

- 2 cloves garlic, minced
- Zest and juice of 1 lemon
- Salt and pepper to taste
- Chopped fresh parsley for garnish

Directions:

1. Season turkey cutlets with salt and pepper.
2. Take a skillet, heat olive oil over medium-high heat. Add ground garlic and cook for 1 minute.
3. Add turkey cutlets to the skillet and cook for 5-7 minutes per side or until cooked through.
4. Sprinkle lemon zest over the turkey cutlets and squeeze lemon juice on top.
5. Garnish with chopped parsley before serving.

Nutrition Information (per serving):

Calories: 280, Protein: 35g, Fat: 14g, Carbohydrates: 3g, Fiber: 1g

Chicken and Spinach Quesadillas

Servings: 2

Prep Time: 10 minutes

Cook Time: 10 minutes

Ingredients:

- 2 whole wheat tortillas
- 1 cup cooked chicken, shredded
- 1 cup fresh spinach leaves
- 1/2 cup shredded low-fat mozzarella cheese
- Cooking spray

Directions:

1. Place one tortilla on a flat surface. Spread shredded chicken, spinach leaves, and shredded mozzarella cheese on half of the tortilla.
2. Wrap the tortilla in half to cover the filling.
3. Put a skillet over medium heat and lightly coat with cooking spray.
4. Lay the quesadilla in the skillet and cook for 3-4 minutes on each side till it turns golden brown and cheese is melted.
5. Remove from heat and let it cool for a minute before slicing into wedges.
6. Serve warm with a side of low-fat sour cream or salsa.

Nutrition Information (per serving):

Calories: 320, Protein: 25g, Fat: 10g, Carbohydrates: 30g, Fiber: 5g

Turkey and Brown Rice Casserole

Servings: 2-3

Prep Time: 15 minutes

Cook Time: 40 minutes

Ingredients:

- 1 cup cooked turkey, shredded
- 1 cup cooked brown rice
- 1/2 cup low-sodium chicken broth
- 1/2 cup carrots, diced
- 1/2 cup zucchini, diced
- 1/2 cup bell peppers, diced
- 1/4 teaspoon dried thyme
- Salt and pepper to taste

Directions:

1. Preset the oven to 375°F (190°C).
2. Take a bowl, mix together the shredded turkey, cooked brown rice, diced carrots, zucchini, bell peppers, dried thyme, salt, and pepper.
3. Place the mixture in a baking dish and pour the chicken broth over it.
4. Wrap the dish with foil and bake for 30-35 minutes until vegetables are tender.

5. Reduce the foil and bake for an additional 5-10 minutes for a golden top.
6. Allow it to cool slightly before serving.

Calories: 250, Protein: 20g, Carbohydrates: 30g, Fat: 5g, Fiber: 4g

Balsamic Glazed Chicken Breasts

Servings: 2

Prep Time: 10 minutes

Cook Time: 20 minutes

Ingredients:

- 2 boneless, skinless chicken breasts
- 2 tablespoons balsamic vinegar
- 1 tablespoon honey
- 1 teaspoon olive oil
- 1/2 teaspoon garlic powder
- Salt and pepper to taste

Directions:

1. Preset the oven to 400°F (200°C).
2. In a bowl, mix balsamic vinegar, honey, olive oil, garlic powder, salt, and pepper.
3. Put down the chicken breasts in a baking dish and brush the balsamic mixture over them.
4. Bake for 18-20 minutes till the chicken is cooked through, occasionally brushing more glaze during cooking.
5. Let it rest for a few minutes before serving.

Nutrition Information (per serving):

Calories: 220, Protein: 25g, Carbohydrates: 8g, Fat: 8g, Fiber: 0.5g

Turkey and Vegetable Skillet

Servings: 2

Prep Time: 10 minutes

Cook Time: 15 minutes

Ingredients:

- 1 cup cooked turkey, chopped
- 1 cup mixed vegetables (bell peppers, broccoli, carrots)
- 1 tablespoon olive oil
- 1/2 teaspoon dried basil
- 1/2 teaspoon paprika
- Salt and pepper to taste

Directions:

1. Put in olive oil in a skillet over medium heat.
2. Add mixed vegetables and sauté until slightly tender.
3. Add chopped turkey, dried basil, paprika, salt, and pepper. Cook for another 5-7 minutes until heated through.
4. Remove from heat and serve warm.

Nutrition Information (per serving):

Calories: 230, Protein: 20g, Carbohydrates: 10g, Fat: 12g, Fiber: 4g

Honey Mustard Grilled Chicken

Servings: 2

Prep Time: 5 minutes

Cook Time: 15 minutes

Ingredients:

- 2 boneless, skinless chicken breasts
- 2 tablespoons honey
- 2 tablespoons Dijon mustard
- 1 tablespoon olive oil
- 1 teaspoon lemon juice
- Salt and pepper to taste

1. Preheat the grill to medium-high heat.
2. In a bowl, mix honey, Dijon mustard, olive oil, lemon juice, salt, and pepper.
3. Brush the mixture over the chicken breasts.
4. Grill the chicken for about 6-8 minutes per side until cooked through, brushing with more sauce while grilling.
5. Allow it to rest for a few minutes before serving.

Nutrition Information (per serving):

Calories: 250, Protein: 25g, Carbohydrates: 15g, Fat: 10g, Fiber: 0.5g

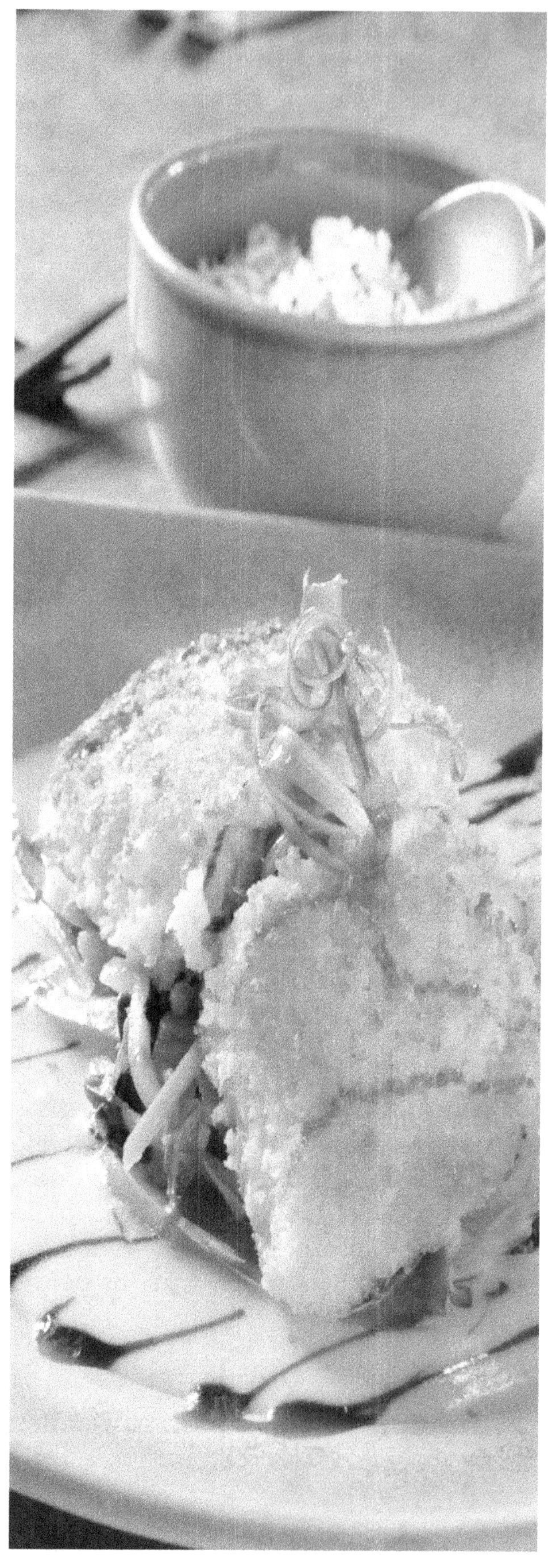

Baked Lemon Herb Cod

Servings: 2

Prep Time: 10 minutes

Cook Time: 15 minutes

Ingredients:

- 2 cod fillets
- 1 tablespoon olive oil
- 1 lemon (juice and zest)
- 1 teaspoon dried thyme
- 1 teaspoon dried rosemary
- Salt and pepper to taste

Directions:

1. Set out your oven to 375°F (190°C).
2. Place the cod fillets on a baking dish lined with parchment paper.
3. Into a small bowl, mix together olive oil, lemon juice, lemon zest, thyme, rosemary, salt, and pepper.
4. Brush the herb mixture over the cod fillets, ensuring they're evenly coated.
5. Bake for about 15 minutes or until the fish flakes easily with a fork.
6. Serve the baked lemon herb cod with steamed vegetables or rice for a complete meal.

Nutrition Information (per serving):

Calories: 180, Protein: 25g, Fat: 7g, Carbohydrates: 2g, Fiber: 1g

Grilled Salmon with Dill

Servings: 2

Prep Time: 10 minutes

Cook Time: 10 minutes

Ingredients:

- 2 salmon fillets
- 1 tablespoon olive oil
- 1 tablespoon fresh dill (chopped)
- 1 garlic clove (minced)
- Salt and pepper to taste

Directions:

1. Preheat your grill to medium heat.
2. Take a small bowl, mix together olive oil, chopped dill, minced garlic, salt, and pepper.
3. Brush the dill mixture onto both sides of the salmon fillets.
4. Place the salmon fillets on the grill and cook for about 4-5 minutes per side or until the fish is cooked through.
5. Serve the grilled salmon with a side of steamed vegetables or a green salad.

Nutrition Information (per serving):

Calories: 250, Protein: 26g, Fat: 15g

Carbohydrates: 1g, Fiber: 0g

Tilapia with Herbed Tomato Salsa

Servings: 2

Prep Time: 15 minutes

Cook Time: 10 minutes

Ingredients:

- 2 tilapia fillets
- 1 cup diced tomatoes
- 2 tablespoons fresh parsley (chopped)
- 1 tablespoon fresh basil (chopped)
- 1 tablespoon olive oil
- 1 garlic clove (minced)
- Salt and pepper to taste

Directions:

1. In a bowl, combine diced tomatoes, parsley, basil, diced

garlic, olive oil, salt, and pepper to make the herbed tomato salsa.
2. Garnish the tilapia fillets with salt and pepper on both sides.
3. Put a skillet over medium heat and lightly oil it.
4. Cook the tilapia fillets for about 3-4 minutes per side or until they easily flake with a fork.
5. Serve the cooked tilapia fillets topped with the herbed tomato salsa.

Calories: 180, Protein: 25g, Fat: 8g, Carbohydrates: 4g, Fiber: 1g

---

Baked Garlic Parmesan Crusted Halibut

Servings: 2

Prep Time: 10 minutes

Cook Time: 15 minutes

Ingredients:

- 2 halibut fillets
- 2 tablespoons grated Parmesan cheese
- 1 tablespoon olive oil
- 2 garlic cloves (minced)
- 1 teaspoon dried parsley
- Salt and pepper to taste

Directions:

1. Set out your oven to 400°F (200°C).
2. Place the halibut fillets on a baking dish lined with parchment paper.
3. Take a small bowl, mix together grated Parmesan, olive oil, minced garlic, dried parsley, salt, and pepper.
4. Spread the Parmesan mixture evenly over the top of each halibut fillet.
5. Bake for about 15 minutes or until the fish is prepared through and flakes easily with a fork.
6. Serve the baked garlic Parmesan crusted halibut with a side of roasted vegetables or quinoa.

Nutrition Information (per serving):

Calories: 220, Protein: 30g, Fat: 10g, Carbohydrates: 1g, Fiber: 0g

---

Lemon Pepper Grilled Tuna Steaks

Serving: 2

Prep Time: 10 minutes

Cook Time: 8-10 minutes

Ingredients:

- 2 tuna steaks (about 6 ounces each)
- 2 tablespoons olive oil
- 1 teaspoon lemon zest
- 1 teaspoon black pepper
- 1/2 teaspoon salt
- 1 tablespoon fresh lemon juice

Directions:

1. Preheat the grill to medium-high heat.
2. Soak up the tuna steaks and place them on a plate.
3. Into a small bowl, mix olive oil, lemon zest, black pepper, salt, and lemon juice to create a marinade.
4. Brush both parts of the tuna steaks with the marinade.
5. Grill the tuna steaks for 4-5 minutes on each side or until desired doneness.
6. Remove from grill and let them rest for a few minutes before serving.

Nutrition Information (per serving):

Calories: 280, Protein: 36g, Fat: 13g, Carbohydrates: 2g, Fiber: 0g

Broiled Lemon Herb Haddock

Serving: 2

Prep Time: 5 minutes

Cook Time: 8-10 minutes

Ingredients:

- 2 haddock fillets (about 6 ounces each)
- 2 tablespoons melted butter or olive oil
- 1 teaspoon lemon juice
- 1/2 teaspoon dried basil
- 1/2 teaspoon dried thyme
- Salt and pepper to taste

Directions:

1. Preheat the broiler in your oven.
2. Place haddock fillets on a baking sheet lined with parchment paper.
3. In a bowl, mix melted butter or olive oil, lemon juice, dried basil, dried thyme, salt, and pepper.
4. Brush the herb mixture over the haddock fillets.
5. Broil for 4-5 minutes on each side up until the fish flakes smoothly with a fork.
6. Serve hot.

Nutrition Information (per serving):

Calories: 220, Protein: 30g, Fat: 9g, Carbohydrates: 0g, Fiber: 0g

Herb-Marinated Grilled Trout

Serving: 2

Prep Time: 15 minutes

Cook Time: 10-12 minutes

Ingredients:

- 2 trout fillets (about 6 ounces each)
- 2 tablespoons olive oil
- 2 cloves garlic, minced
- 1 tablespoon fresh parsley, chopped
- 1 tablespoon fresh thyme, chopped
- Salt and pepper to taste

Directions:

1. Preheat the grill to medium heat.
2. Pat dry the trout fillets and place them on a plate.
3. Take a bowl, mix olive oil, minced garlic, chopped parsley, chopped thyme, salt, and pepper to create a marinade.
4. Brush both sides of the trout fillets with the marinade.
5. Grill the trout fillets for 5-6 minutes on each side or until cooked through.
6. Remove from grill and let them rest for a few minutes before serving.

Nutrition Information (per serving):

Calories: 260, Protein: 36g, Fat: 12g, Carbohydrates: 1g, Fiber: 0g

Salmon Salad Stuffed Avocado

Serving: 2

Prep Time: 15 minutes

Cook Time: 0 minutes

Ingredients:

- 1 ripe avocado, halved and pitted
- 1 can (6 ounces) salmon, drained
- 2 tablespoons Greek yogurt or mayonnaise
- 1 tablespoon lemon juice
- 2 tablespoons finely chopped red onion
- Salt and pepper to taste
- Optional: chopped fresh herbs like dill or parsley for garnish

Directions:

1. In a bowl, combine drained salmon, Greek yogurt or mayonnaise, lemon

juice, chopped red onion, salt, and pepper.
2. Mix well until all ingredients are combined.
3. Spoon the salmon salad mixture into the avocado halves.
4. Garnish with chopped fresh herbs if desired.
5. Serve immediately.

<u>Nutrition Information (per serving):</u>

Calories: 320, Protein: 20g, Fat: 22g, Carbohydrates: 12g, Fiber: 8g

Baked Mediterranean Style Sardines

Servings: 2

Prep Time: 15 minutes

Cook Time: 20 minutes

<u>Ingredients:</u>

- 4 fresh sardines, cleaned and gutted
- 2 tablespoons olive oil
- 2 cloves garlic, minced
- 1 teaspoon dried oregano
- 1 teaspoon dried thyme
- 1 lemon, thinly sliced
- Salt and pepper to taste

<u>Directions:</u>

1. Put your oven to 375°F (190°C).
2. Rinse the sardines under cold water and pat them dry with paper towels.
3. Place a small bowl, mix together olive oil, minced garlic, oregano, and thyme.
4. Place the sardines on a baking sheet lined with parchment paper. Brush them generously with the olive oil mixture.
5. Garnish the sardines with salt and pepper, and place lemon slices on top.

6. Bake in the preset oven for about 15-20 minutes until the sardines are cooked through and tender.
7. Serve the baked sardines with a side of steamed vegetables or a simple salad.

<u>Nutrition Information: (per serving)</u>

Calories: 220 kcal, Protein: 20g, Fat: 14g, Carbohydrates: 2g, Fiber: 1g

Lemon Garlic Shrimp Skewers

Servings: 2

Prep Time: 10 minutes

Cook Time: 6 minutes

<u>Ingredients:</u>

- 12 large shrimp, peeled and deveined
- 2 cloves garlic, minced
- 2 tablespoons olive oil
- Zest and juice of 1 lemon
- Salt and pepper to taste
- Wooden skewers, soaked in water

<u>Directions:</u>

1. Preheat your grill or grill pan over medium heat.
2. In a bowl, mix together minced garlic, olive oil, lemon zest, lime juice, salt, and pepper.
3. Thread the shrimp onto the rinsed wooden skewers.
4. Brush the shrimp with the prepared garlic and lemon marinade.
5. Grill the skewers for about 2-3 minutes on each side up until the shrimp turn pink and opaque.
6. Serve the lemon garlic shrimp skewers with a side of quinoa or steamed rice.

<u>Nutrition Information: (per serving)</u>

Calories: 180 kcal, Protein: 22g, Fat: 9g, Carbohydrates: 3g, Fiber: 1g

Herb-Roasted Mackerel

Servings: 2

Prep Time: 10 minutes

Cook Time: 15 minutes

Ingredients:

- 2 mackerel fillets
- 2 tablespoons olive oil
- 1 teaspoon dried rosemary
- 1 teaspoon dried thyme
- 1 teaspoon paprika
- Salt and pepper to taste
- Lemon wedges for serving

Directions:

1. Preset your oven to 400°F (200°C).
2. Lay off the mackerel fillets on a baking sheet lined with parchment paper.
3. Take a small bowl, mix together olive oil, rosemary, thyme, paprika, salt, and pepper.
4. Brush the herb and spice mixture onto the mackerel fillets.
5. Roast in the oven for about 12-15 minutes until the mackerel is cooked through and flakes easily with a fork.
6. Serve the herb-roasted mackerel with lemon wedges and a side of steamed vegetables.

Nutrition Information: (per serving)

Calories: 250 kcal, Protein: 20g, Fat: 18g, Carbohydrates: 0g, Fiber: 0g

Crispy Baked Dijon Mustard Catfish

Servings: 2

Prep Time: 10 minutes

Cook Time: 20 minutes

Ingredients:

- 2 catfish fillets
- 2 tablespoons Dijon mustard
- 2 tablespoons breadcrumbs
- 1 tablespoon olive oil
- 1 teaspoon paprika
- Salt and pepper to taste
- Fresh parsley for garnish

Directions:

1. Place your oven to 375°F (190°C). Line a baking sheet with parchment paper.
2. Pat dry the catfish fillets with paper towels and place them on the prepared baking sheet.
3. Into a small bowl, mix together Dijon mustard, breadcrumbs, olive oil, paprika, salt, and pepper.
4. Spread the mustard mixture evenly over the catfish fillets.
5. Cook in the warmed up oven for approximately 15-20 minutes until the catfish is crispy and cooked through.
6. Garnish with fresh parsley before serving.

Nutrition Information: (per serving)

Calories: 230 kcal, Protein: 25g, Fat: 10g, Carbohydrates: 4g, Fiber: 1g

Grilled Swordfish with Mango Salsa

Servings: 2

Prep Time: 15 minutes

Cook Time: 10 minutes

Ingredients:

- 2 swordfish fillets (about 6 ounces each)
- Salt and pepper to taste
- For Mango Salsa:
- 1 ripe mango, diced

- 1/4 cup red onion, finely chopped
- 1/4 cup fresh cilantro, chopped
- 1 jalapeño pepper, seeded and finely chopped
- Juice of 1 lime
- Salt to taste

Directions:

1. Preheat grill to medium-high heat.
2. Season swordfish fillets with salt and pepper.
3. Grill swordfish for about 4-5 minutes per side or until cooked through.
4. In a bowl, combine diced mango, red onion, cilantro, jalapeño, lime juice, and salt to make the salsa.
5. Serve grilled swordfish topped with mango salsa.

Nutrition Information (per serving):

Calories: 280, Protein: 32g, Fat: 8g, Carbohydrates: 20g, Fiber: 3g

Baked Orange Glazed Mahi Mahi

Servings: 2

Prep Time: 10 minutes

Cook Time: 20 minutes

Ingredients:

- 2 mahi mahi fillets (about 5-6 ounces each)
- Salt and pepper to taste
- 1/4 cup orange juice
- 2 tablespoons honey
- 1 tablespoon low-sodium soy sauce
- 1 teaspoon grated fresh ginger
- 1 garlic clove, minced

Directions:

1. Preheat oven to 375°F (190°C).
2. Garnish the mahi mahi fillets with salt and pepper and lay them in a baking dish.
3. Take a bowl, mix together orange juice, honey, soy sauce, ginger, and garlic.
4. Pour the orange glaze over the fish fillets.
5. Bake for 15-20 minutes or until the fish is prepared through and flakes easily with a fork.

Nutrition Information (per serving):

Calories: 240, Protein: 34g, Fat: 3g, Carbohydrates: 21g, Fiber: 1g

Grilled Lemon Garlic Sea Bass

Servings: 2

Prep Time: 10 minutes

Cook Time: 12 minutes

Ingredients:

- 2 sea bass fillets (about 5-6 ounces each)
- Salt and pepper to taste
- Juice of 1 lemon
- 2 garlic cloves, minced
- 2 tablespoons olive oil

Directions:

1. Preheat grill to medium heat.
2. Garnish the sea bass fillets with salt and pepper.
3. Take a small bowl, mix together lemon juice, minced garlic, and olive oil.
4. Brush the lemon garlic mixture over the fish fillets.
5. Grill sea bass for about 5-6 minutes per side or until the fish is cooked through.

Nutrition Information (per serving):

Calories: 290, Protein: 38g, Fat: 14g, Carbohydrates: 2g, Fiber: 0g

Herb-Crusted Baked Snapper

Servings: 2

Prep Time: 15 minutes

Cook Time: 20 minutes

Ingredients:

- 2 snapper fillets (about 6 ounces each)
- Salt and pepper to taste
- 2 tablespoons shredded fresh herbs (parsley, thyme, rosemary)
- 2 tablespoons breadcrumbs (use gluten-free if needed)
- 1 tablespoon olive oil

Directions:

1. Preheat oven to 400°F (200°C).
2. Garnish the snapper fillets with salt and pepper and place them on a baking sheet.
3. In a bowl, combine chopped herbs, breadcrumbs, and olive oil to form a crumb mixture.
4. Press the herb and breadcrumb mixture onto the top of each snapper fillet.
5. Cook it for 15-20 minutes or till the fish is fixed and the crust is golden.

Nutrition Information (per serving):

Calories: 260, Protein: 36g, Fat: 9g, Carbohydrates: 7g, Fiber: 1g

Cajun-Style Baked Redfish

Servings: 2

Prep Time: 10 minutes

Cook Time: 20 minutes

Ingredients:

- 2 redfish fillets
- 1 tablespoon olive oil
- 1 teaspoon paprika
- 1/2 teaspoon garlic powder
- 1/2 teaspoon onion powder
- 1/4 teaspoon cayenne pepper (adjust to taste)
- Salt and pepper to taste
- Lemon wedges (for serving)
- Chopped fresh parsley (for garnish, optional)

Directions:

1. Put your oven to 375°F (190°C). Spread out a baking sheet with parchment paper or lightly grease it.
2. Pat dry the redfish fillets with paper towels. Place them on the prepared baking sheet.
3. Into a small bowl, mix together olive oil, paprika, garlic powder, onion powder, cayenne pepper, salt, and pepper.
4. Brush the spice mixture evenly over the redfish fillets.
5. Cook in the warm oven for about 15-20 minutes or until the fish is prepared through and flakes easily with a fork.
6. Once done, remove from the oven. Squeeze out fresh lemon juice over the fish and garnish with chopped parsley if desired. Serve warm.

Nutrition Information (per serving):

Calories: 250, Protein: 30g, Fat: 12g, Carbohydrates: 2g, Fiber: 1g

Poached Cod with Herbed Butter Sauce

Servings: 2

Prep Time: 5 minutes

Cook Time: 15 minutes

Ingredients:

- 2 cod fillets
- 2 tablespoons unsalted butter

- 1 tablespoon chopped fresh herbs (parsley, dill, or thyme)
- Salt and pepper to taste
- Lemon wedges (for serving)

1. In a shallow skillet or saucepan, bring water to a gentle simmer.
2. Place the cod fillets into the simmering water and let them cook for about 8-10 minutes until they are hazy and easily flake with a fork.
3. In another small saucepan, melt the butter over low heat. Add the minced fresh herbs, salt, and pepper. Stir well.
4. Once the cod fillets are cooked, carefully remove them from the poaching liquid and place them on serving plates.
5. Spoon the herbed butter sauce over the cod fillets. Serve with lemon wedges on the side.

Nutrition Information (per serving):

Calories: 280, Protein: 25g, Fat: 18g, Carbohydrates: 0g, Fiber: 0g

Baked Teriyaki Glazed Trout

Servings: 2

Prep Time: 10 minutes

Cook Time: 15 minutes

Ingredients:

- 2 trout fillets
- 3 tablespoons low-sodium teriyaki sauce
- 1 tablespoon honey
- 1 teaspoon minced ginger
- 1 teaspoon minced garlic
- Sesame seeds (for garnish, optional)
- Sliced green onions (for garnish, optional)

Directions:

1. Place your oven to 400°F (200°C). Lay a baking paper with parchment paper or lightly grease it.
2. Take a small bowl, mix together the teriyaki sauce, honey, minced ginger, and minced garlic.
3. Lay the trout fillets on the prepared baking sheet.
4. Brush the teriyaki mixture evenly over the trout fillets.
5. Cook it in the preheated oven for about 12-15 minutes or until the fish is cooked through and easily flakes with a fork.
6. Once done, remove from the oven. Drizzle sesame seeds and sliced green onions over the trout if desired. Serve hot.

Nutrition Information (per serving):

Calories: 260, Protein: 25g, Fat: 10g, Carbohydrates: 15g, Fiber: 0g

Pan-Seared Lemon Pepper Tilapia

Servings: 2

Prep Time: 5 minutes

Cook Time: 10 minutes

Ingredients:

- 2 tilapia fillets
- 1 tablespoon olive oil
- 1 teaspoon lemon pepper seasoning
- 1/2 teaspoon garlic powder
- Salt to taste
- Lemon wedges (for serving)
- Fresh chopped parsley (for garnish, optional)

Directions:

1. Dry up the tilapia fillets with paper towels and garnish both sides with

lemon pepper seasoning, garlic powder, and salt.

2. Set out olive oil in a non-stick skillet over medium heat.

3. Once the skillet is hot, place the seasoned tilapia fillets in the pan.

4. Sear the fish for about 3-4 minutes on each side until golden brown and cooked through.

5. Once done, remove the tilapia from the skillet and transfer to serving plates.

6. Set with lemon wedges and garnish with fresh chopped parsley if desired.

Nutrition Information (per serving):

Calories: 220, Protein: 30g, Fat: 10g, Carbohydrates: 1g, Fiber: 0g

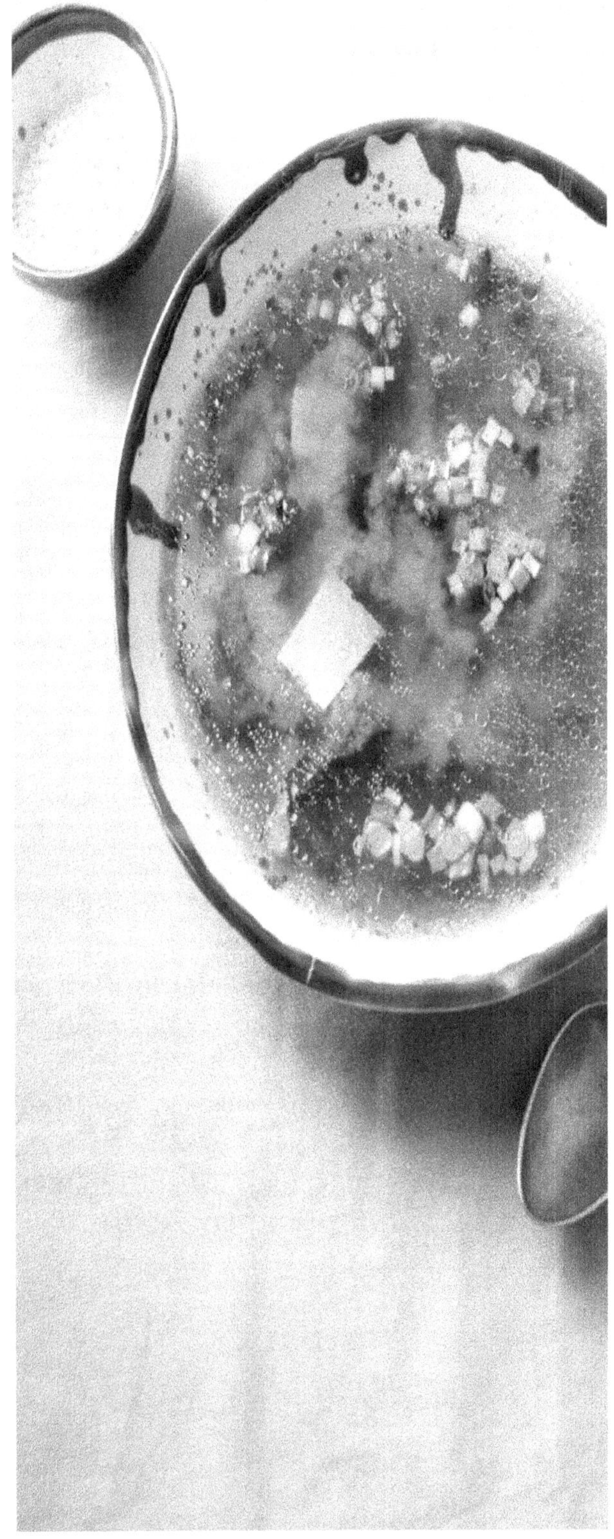

Vegetable Soup

Servings: 2

Prep Time: 15 minutes

Cook Time: 25 minutes

Ingredients:

- 2 cups low-sodium vegetable broth
- 1 cup mixed vegetables (carrots, celery, bell peppers, zucchini)
- 1 small onion, diced
- 2 cloves garlic, minced
- 1 tablespoon olive oil
- Salt and pepper to taste
- 1 teaspoon dry herbs (such as thyme or oregano)

Directions:

1. Put olive oil in a pot over medium heat. Add diced onion and garlic, sauté until fragrant.
2. Add mixed vegetables and sauté for 5 minutes.
3. Lay in the vegetable broth and bring to a boil.
4. Decrease the heat and simmer for 15-20 minutes until vegetables are tender.
5. Season with salt, pepper, and dried herbs.
6. Serve hot.

Nutrition Information (per serving):

Calories: 120, Total Fat: 5g, Sodium: 300mg, Carbohydrates: 18g, Fiber: 5g, Protein: 3g

Tomato Basil Soup

Servings: 2

Prep Time: 10 minutes

Cook Time: 25 minutes

Ingredients:

- 1 can (14 oz) low-sodium diced tomatoes
- 1 cup low-sodium vegetable broth
- 1 small onion, chopped
- 2 cloves garlic, minced
- 1 tablespoon olive oil
- 2 tablespoons chopped fresh basil
- Salt and pepper to taste

Directions:

1. Put olive oil in a pot over medium heat. Add carved onion and garlic, cook until soft.
2. Add diced tomatoes (with their juices) and vegetable broth. Bring to a boil.
3. Reduce heat and simmer for 15-20 minutes.
4. Stir in fresh basil. Use an immersion grinder or regular blender to blend the soup until smooth.
5. Season with salt and pepper.
6. Serve warm.

Nutrition Information (per serving):

Calories: 100, Total Fat: 5g, Sodium: 250mg, Carbohydrates: 12g, Fiber: 3g, Protein: 2g

Butternut Squash Soup

Servings: 2

Prep Time: 15 minutes

Cook Time: 30 minutes

Ingredients:

- 2 cups cubed butternut squash
- 1 small onion, chopped
- 2 cloves garlic, minced
- 2 cups low-sodium vegetable broth
- 1 tablespoon olive oil
- 1 teaspoon ground cinnamon
- Salt and pepper to taste

Directions:

1. Put olive oil in a pot over medium heat. Add chopped out onion and garlic, cook until translucent.
2. Add butternut squash cubes and vegetable broth. Bring to a boil.
3. Decrease the heat and simmer for 20-25 minutes until squash is tender.
4. Use an immersion grinder or regular blender to puree the soup until smooth.
5. Stir in ground cinnamon, salt, and pepper.
6. Serve hot.

Nutrition Information (per serving):

Calories: 150, Total Fat: 6g, Sodium: 300mg, Carbohydrates: 22g, Fiber: 5g, Protein: 3g

Minestrone Soup

Servings: 2

Prep Time: 15 minutes

Cook Time: 25 minutes

Ingredients:

- 2 cups low-sodium vegetable broth
- 1 can (14 oz) low-sodium diced tomatoes
- 1/2 cup small- scale pasta (such as elbow or shell pasta)
- 1 cup mixed vegetables (carrots, celery, green beans)
- 1 small onion, chopped
- 2 cloves garlic, minced
- 1 tablespoon olive oil
- 1 teaspoon dried Italian herbs
- Salt and pepper to taste

Directions:

1. Put olive oil in a pot over medium heat. Add diced onion and garlic, cook until softened.
2. Add mixed vegetables and sauté for 5 minutes.
3. Spread in vegetable broth and diced tomatoes (with their juices).
4. Add pasta and simmer down for 10-12 minutes until pasta is cooked.
5. Stir in dried Italian herbs, salt, and pepper.
6. Serve warm.

Nutrition Information (per serving):

Calories: 180, Total Fat: 5g, Sodium: 350mg, Carbohydrates: 30g, Fiber: 6g, Protein: 5g

Lentil Soup

Serving: 2

Prep Time: 10 minutes

Cook Time: 30 minutes

Ingredients:

- 1 cup red lentils, rinsed
- 4 cups low-sodium chicken or vegetable broth
- 1 carrot, diced
- 1 celery stalk, diced
- 1 small onion, finely chopped
- 2 cloves garlic, minced
- 1 teaspoon ground cumin
- 1 teaspoon paprika
- Salt and pepper to taste
- Fresh parsley for garnish (optional)

Directions:

1. In a pot, combine lentils, broth, carrot, celery, onion, garlic, cumin, and paprika.
2. Bring the compound to a boil, then reduce heat and simmer down for 25-30 minutes until lentils are tender.
3. Garnish with salt and pepper according to taste.
4. Set out hot, garnished with fresh parsley if desired.

Nutrition Information (per serving):

Calories: 280, Total Fat: 1g, Sodium: 480mg, Total Carbohydrates: 50g, Fiber: 18g, Protein: 18g

Chicken and Rice Soup

Serving: 2

Prep Time: 15 minutes

Cook Time: 40 minutes

Ingredients:

- 2 boneless, skinless chicken breasts, diced
- 4 cups low-sodium chicken broth
- 1/2 cup white rice
- 1 carrot, sliced
- 1 celery stalk, sliced
- 1 small onion, finely chopped
- 2 cloves garlic, minced
- 1 bay leaf
- Salt and pepper to taste
- Fresh parsley for garnish (optional)

Directions:

1. In a pot, combine chicken, chicken broth, rice, carrot, celery, onion, garlic, and bay leaf.
2. After a boil, then reduce heat and simmer for 30-35 minutes until chicken is cooked through and rice is tender.
3. Remove the bay leaf, season with salt and pepper according to taste.
4. Set out hot, garnished with fresh parsley if desired.

Nutrition Information (per serving):

Calories: 320, Total Fat: 3g, Sodium: 560mg, Total Carbohydrates: 40g, Fiber: 3g, Protein: 34g

Miso Soup with Tofu and Seaweed

Serving: 2

Prep Time: 10 minutes

Cook Time: 10 minutes

Ingredients:

- 4 cups water
- 2 tablespoons miso paste (preferably white)
- 1 cup firm tofu, diced
- 2 sheets nori seaweed, torn into small pieces
- 2 green onions, thinly sliced

Directions:

1. In a pot, bring water to a gentle simmer.
2. Melt the miso paste in a small amount of hot water, then add it to the pot.
3. Add tofu and nori seaweed, simmer for 5-7 minutes.
4. Stir in green onions.
5. Serve hot.

Nutrition Information (per serving):

Calories: 180, Total Fat: 9g, Sodium: 800mg, Total Carbohydrates: 14g, Fiber: 2g, Protein: 14g

Potato Leek Soup

Serving: 2

Prep Time: 15 minutes

Cook Time: 25 minutes

Ingredients:

- 2 leeks, white and greenish parts only, sliced
- 2 potatoes, peeled and diced
- 3 cups low-sodium chicken or vegetable broth
- 1 tablespoon olive oil

- Salt and pepper to taste
- Fresh chives for garnish (optional)

Directions:

1. Take a pot, heat olive oil over medium heat. Add leeks and sauté until softened.
2. Put potatoes and broth, bring to a boil, then decrease the heat and simmer for 20-25 minutes until potatoes are tender.
3. Use a grinder or transfer to a blender to puree the soup until smooth.
4. Garnish with salt and pepper according to taste.
5. Serve hot, garnished with fresh chives if desired.

Nutrition Information (per serving):

Calories: 240, Total Fat: 4g, Sodium: 480mg, Total Carbohydrates: 50g, Fiber: 6g, Protein: 5g

---

Pumpkin Soup

Servings: 2

Prep Time: 10 minutes

Cook Time: 25 minutes

Ingredients:

- 2 cups diced pumpkin
- 1 small onion, chopped
- 2 cloves garlic, minced
- 2 cups low-sodium chicken or vegetable broth
- 1/2 teaspoon ground cinnamon
- Salt and pepper to taste
- 1 tablespoon olive oil

Directions:

1. Put olive oil in a pot over medium heat. Add chopped onions and garlic, sauté until translucent.
2. Add diced pumpkin to the pot and stir for a few minutes.
3. Pour in the broth, add cinnamon, salt, and pepper. After a boil, then decrease the heat and simmer for 20-25 minutes until pumpkin is tender.
4. Let the compound cool slightly, then blend until smooth using an grinder or regular blender.
5. Reheat if necessary and serve warm.

Nutrition Information (per serving):

Calories: 120, Total Fat: 5g, Carbohydrates: 20g, Fiber: 4g, Protein: 2g

---

Vegetable Barley Stew

Servings: 2

Prep Time: 15 minutes

Cook Time: 40 minutes

Ingredients:

- 1/2 cup pearl barley
- 2 cups low-sodium vegetable broth
- 1 cup mixed vegetables (carrots, celery, bell peppers), chopped
- 1 small onion, diced
- 2 cloves garlic, minced
- 1 tablespoon olive oil
- 1 teaspoon dried thyme
- Salt and pepper to taste

Directions:

1. Put olive oil in a pot over medium heat. Add diced onions, minced garlic, and chopped vegetables. Sauté until softened.
2. Add barley, vegetable broth, thyme, salt, and pepper. After a boil, then decrease the heat and simmer for 35-40 minutes until barley is tender.

3. Adjust seasoning if needed and serve hot.

Nutrition Information (per serving):

Calories: 250, Total Fat: 6g, Carbohydrates: 45g, Fiber: 9g, Protein: 6g

Spinach and White Bean Soup

Servings: 2

Prep Time: 10 minutes

Cook Time: 20 minutes

Ingredients:

- 2 cups fresh spinach leaves
- 1 can (15 oz) white beans, drained and rinsed
- 1 small onion, chopped
- 2 cloves garlic, minced
- 3 cups low-sodium chicken or vegetable broth
- 1 tablespoon olive oil
- 1 teaspoon dried basil
- Salt and pepper to taste

Directions:

1. Put olive oil in a pot over medium heat. Add chopped onions and minced garlic, sauté until fragrant.
2. Lay spinach leaves to the pot and cook until wilted.
3. Stir in white beans, broth, dried basil, salt, and pepper. Bring to a simmer down and cook for 15-20 minutes.
4. Blend a portion of the soup if desired for a creamier texture.
5. Adjust seasoning and serve warm.

Nutrition Information (per serving):

Calories: 220, Total Fat: 6g, Carbohydrates: 30g, Fiber: 8g, Protein: 12g

Broccoli and Cauliflower Soup

Servings: 2

Prep Time: 15 minutes

Cook Time: 25 minutes

Ingredients:

- 1 cup broccoli florets
- 1 cup cauliflower florets
- 1 small onion, chopped
- 2 cloves garlic, minced
- 2 cups low-sodium chicken or vegetable broth
- 1 tablespoon olive oil
- 1/2 teaspoon dried thyme
- Salt and pepper to taste

Directions:

1. Put olive oil in a pot over medium heat. Add chopped onions and minced garlic, sauté until onions are translucent.
2. Add broccoli, cauliflower, broth, dried thyme, salt, and pepper. After a boil, then decrease the heat and simmer down for 20-25 minutes until vegetables are tender.
3. Let it cool a bit, then blend until smooth using an grinder or regular blender.
4. Reheat if needed and serve hot.

Nutrition Information (per serving):

Calories: 150, Total Fat: 6g, Carbohydrates: 20g, Fiber: 6g, Protein: 8g

Corn Chowder

Servings: 2

Prep Time: 10 minutes

Cook Time: 25 minutes

Ingredients:

- 1 cup frozen corn kernels

- 1 small potato, diced
- 1 cup low-fat milk or almond milk
- 1 cup low-sodium chicken or vegetable broth
- 1 tablespoon olive oil
- 1/2 onion, chopped
- 1/4 teaspoon dried thyme
- Salt and pepper to taste

Directions:

1. Put olive oil in a pot over medium heat. Add chopped onion and sauté until translucent.
2. Add diced potato, corn kernels, thyme, salt, and pepper. Stir for 2-3 minutes.
3. Lay in the broth and bring it to a gentle boil. Reduce heat and simmer down until the potatoes are tender (around 15-20 minutes).
4. Blend half of the soup until smooth, then return it to the pot. Stir in the milk and let it warm through for a few minutes. Adjust seasoning if needed.
5. Serve warm.

Nutrition Information (per serving):

Calories: 250, Protein: 6g, Carbohydrates: 40g, Fat: 8g, Fiber: 5g

Ginger Carrot Soup

Servings: 2

Prep Time: 10 minutes

Cook Time: 25 minutes

Ingredients:

- 4 large carrots, peeled and chopped
- 1 small onion, chopped
- 1 tablespoon fresh ginger, grated
- 2 cups low-sodium chicken or vegetable broth
- 1 cup water

- 1 tablespoon olive oil
- Salt and pepper to taste
- Fresh cilantro for garnish (optional)

Directions:

1. Put olive oil in a pot over medium heat. Add chopped onion and grated ginger. Sauté until fragrant.
2. Add chopped carrots, broth, water, salt, and pepper. After a boil, then reduce the heat to a simmer. Lid and cook until carrots are tender (about 20 minutes).
3. Mix the soup until smooth using an immersion blender or regular blender.
4. Serve hot, seasoned with fresh cilantro if desired.

Nutrition Information (per serving):

Calories: 180, Protein: 4g, Carbohydrates: 25g, Fat: 7g, Fiber: 7g

Split Pea Soup

Servings: 2

Prep Time: 10 minutes

Cook Time: 45 minutes

Ingredients:

- 1 cup dried split peas, rinsed
- 1 small onion, chopped
- 2 carrots, chopped
- 2 cups low-sodium chicken or vegetable broth
- 2 cups water
- 1 bay leaf
- 1 tablespoon olive oil
- Salt and pepper to taste

Directions:

1. Put olive oil in a pot over medium heat. Add chopped onion and sauté until soft.

2. Add split peas, carrots, bay leaf, broth, and water. After a boil, then decrease the heat to low. Cover and simmer for about 40-45 minutes until peas are tender.
3. Remove the bay leaf. Use an immersion grinder or regular blender to puree half of the soup until smooth.
4. Season with salt and pepper. Serve hot.

Nutrition Information (per serving):

Calories: 280, Protein: 16g, Carbohydrates: 45g, Fat: 4g, Fiber: 18g

Vegetable Quinoa Chili

Servings: 2

Prep Time: 15 minutes

Cook Time: 30 minutes

Ingredients:

- 1/2 cup quinoa, rinsed
- 1 can (15 oz) low-sodium black beans, drained and rinsed
- 1 can (14 oz) diced tomatoes
- 1 cup low-sodium vegetable broth
- 1 cup mixed vegetables (bell peppers, corn, zucchini)
- 1/2 onion, chopped
- 1 clove garlic, minced
- 1 teaspoon chili powder
- 1/2 teaspoon cumin
- Salt and pepper to taste
- 1 tablespoon olive oil
- Fresh cilantro for garnish (optional)

Directions:

1. Take a pot, heat olive oil over medium heat. Add chopped onion and garlic, sauté until fragrant.
2. Add mixed vegetables, quinoa, black beans, diced tomatoes (with juices), vegetable broth, chili powder, cumin, salt, and pepper. Stir well.
3. After a boil, then reduce heat to low. Cover and simmer for about 20-25 minutes until quinoa is cooked and vegetables are tender.
4. Adjust seasoning if needed.
5. Serve hot, seasoned with fresh cilantro if desired.

Nutrition Information (per serving):

Calories: 380, Protein: 16g, Carbohydrates: 65g, Fat: 7g, Fiber: 16g

Chickpea and Vegetable Stew

Serving: 2

Prep Time: 10 minutes

Cook Time: 25 minutes

Ingredients:

- 1 can (15 oz) chickpeas, drained off and rinsed
- 2 cups mixed vegetables (carrots, bell peppers, zucchini), chopped
- 1 onion, diced
- 2 cloves garlic, minced
- 2 cups low-sodium vegetable broth
- 1 teaspoon dried thyme
- Salt and pepper to taste
- 2 tablespoons olive oil

Directions:

1. Into a pot, heat olive oil over medium heat. Add diced onions and minced garlic. Sauté until onions turn translucent.
2. Add mixed vegetables and chickpeas. Cook for 5 minutes, stirring occasionally.
3. Pour in the vegetable broth, add dried thyme, salt, and pepper. Bring to a simmer down and cook for 15-20 minutes until vegetables are tender.

4. Serve warm and enjoy this comforting stew.

Nutrition Information (per serving):

Calories: 280, Protein: 9g, Carbohydrates: 40g, Fat: 9g, Fiber: 10g

Egg Drop Soup

Serving: 2

Prep Time: 5 minutes

Cook Time: 10 minutes

Ingredients:

- 4 cups low-sodium chicken or vegetable broth
- 2 eggs, beaten
- 2 green onions, thinly sliced
- 1 teaspoon ginger, grated
- Salt and pepper to taste

Directions:

1. Take a pot, bring the broth to a gentle boil over medium heat.
2. Gently pour the beaten eggs into the simmering broth while stirring gently in a circular motion.
3. Add grated ginger, salt, and pepper. Prepare for 1-2 minutes until the eggs are cooked through.
4. Season with sliced green onions and serve hot.

Nutrition Information (per serving):

Calories: 70, Protein: 6g, Carbohydrates: 3g, Fat: 4g, Fiber: 0g

Cabbage and Potato Stew

Serving: 2

Prep Time: 10 minutes

Cook Time: 20 minutes

Ingredients:

- 2 cups cabbage, shredded
- 2 potatoes, diced
- 1 onion, chopped
- 2 cloves garlic, minced
- 2 cups low-sodium vegetable broth
- 1 teaspoon paprika
- Salt and pepper to taste
- 2 tablespoons olive oil

Directions:

1. Put olive oil in a pot over medium heat. Add chopped onions and minced garlic. Sauté until fragrant.
2. Add diced potatoes and shredded cabbage. Cook for 5 minutes, stirring occasionally.
3. Pour in the vegetable broth, add paprika, salt, and pepper. Simmer down for 15 minutes or until the potatoes are tender.
4. Serve this hearty stew warm.

Nutrition Information (per serving):

Calories: 230, Protein: 4g, Carbohydrates: 35g, Fat: 9g, Fiber: 6g

Bean and Kale Soup

Serving: 2

Prep Time: 15 minutes

Cook Time: 25 minutes

Ingredients:

- 1 can (15 oz) white beans, drained and rinsed
- 2 cups kale, chopped
- 1 onion, diced

- 2 cloves garlic, minced
- 2 cups low-sodium vegetable broth
- 1 teaspoon dried thyme
- Salt and pepper to taste
- 2 tablespoons olive oil

Directions:

1. Into a pot, heat olive oil over medium heat. Add diced onions and minced garlic. Sauté until onions are soft.
2. Add carved kale and cook until slightly wilted.
3. Add white beans, vegetable broth, dried thyme, salt, and pepper. Bring to a simmer down and cook for 20 minutes.
4. Serve this nutritious soup hot.

Nutrition Information (per serving):

Calories: 270, Protein: 10g, Carbohydrates: 38g, Fat: 8g, Fiber: 10g

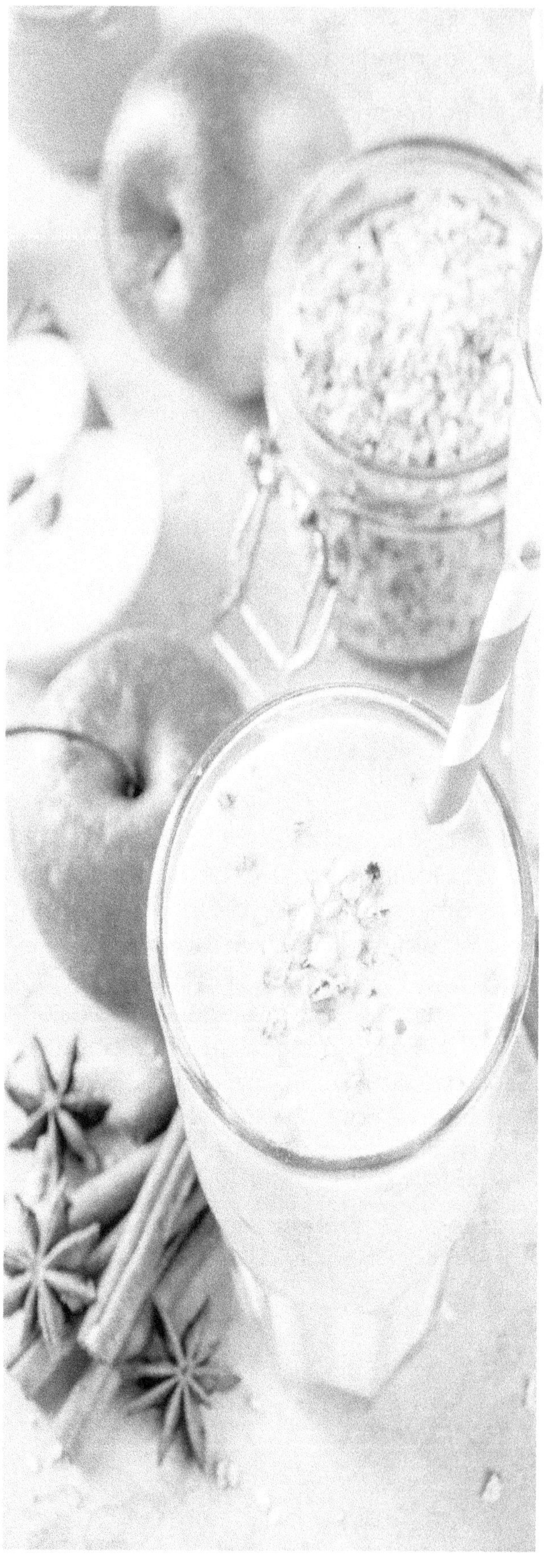

Smoothies

Berry Blast Smoothie

Serving: 1-2

Prep Time: 5 minutes

Ingredients:

- 1 cup mixed berries (strawberries, blueberries, raspberries)
- 1 ripe banana
- 1/2 cup plain Greek yogurt
- 1/2 cup almond milk (unsweetened)
- 1 tablespoon honey (optional)

Directions:

1. Wash the berries thoroughly.
2. Peel off the banana and break it into chunks.
3. Combine all the ingredients in a blender.
4. Blend until smooth and creamy.
5. Serve immediately.

Nutrition Information (per serving):

Calories: 150, Protein: 6g, Fat: 3g, Carbohydrates: 28g, Fiber: 5g

Green Power Smoothie

Serving: 1-2

Prep Time: 7 minutes

Ingredients:

- 1 cup fresh spinach
- 1 ripe avocado
- 1 green apple, cored and chopped
- 1/2 cucumber, peeled and chopped
- 1/2 cup coconut water
- Juice of 1/2 lemon

Directions:

1. Wash the spinach and other produce thoroughly.
2. Peel and pit the avocado.
3. Combine all the ingredients in a blender.
4. Blend until smooth and creamy.
5. Pour into glasses and serve chilled.

Nutrition Information (per serving):

Calories: 200, Protein: 4g, Fat: 12g, Carbohydrates: 23g, Fiber: 10g

Tropical Paradise Smoothie

Serving: 1-2

Prep Time: 5 minutes

Ingredients:

- 1 cup frozen pineapple chunks
- 1 ripe mango, peeled and chopped
- 1/2 cup coconut milk (unsweetened)
- 1/2 cup plain Greek yogurt
- 1 tablespoon chia seeds (optional)

Directions:

1. Combine all the ingredients in a blender.
2. Blend until smooth and creamy.
3. Put more coconut milk if a thinner consistency is desired.
4. Serve immediately.

Nutrition Information (per serving):

Calories: 220, Protein: 7g, Fat: 8g, Carbohydrates: 32g, Fiber: 6g

Banana Almond Smoothie

Serving: 1-2

Prep Time: 5 minutes

Ingredients:

- 2 ripe bananas
- 1/4 cup almond butter
- 1/2 teaspoon ground cinnamon

- 1 cup almond milk (unsweetened)
- Ice cubes (optional)

Directions:

1. Peel off the bananas and break them into chunks.
2. Combine bananas, almond butter, cinnamon, almond milk, and ice cubes (if using) in a blender.
3. Blend until smooth and creamy.
4. Pour into glasses and serve immediately.

Nutrition Information (per serving):

Calories: 250, Protein: 5g, Fat: 15g, Carbohydrates: 28g, Fiber: 6g

Peachy Keen Smoothie

Serving: 1-2

Prep Time: 5 minutes

Ingredients:

- 2 ripe peaches, pitted and chopped
- 1/2 cup plain Greek yogurt
- 1/2 cup almond milk (unsweetened)
- 1 tablespoon honey (optional)
- 1/2 teaspoon vanilla extract

Directions:

1. Wash and chop the peaches.
2. Combine peaches, Greek yogurt, almond milk, honey, and vanilla extract in a blender.
3. Blend until smooth and creamy.
4. Taste and adjust sweetness if needed.
5. Serve immediately.

Nutrition Information (per serving):

Calories: 180, Protein: 7g, Fat: 3g, Carbohydrates: 32g, Fiber: 4g

Avocado Spinach Smoothie

Servings: 1-2

Prep Time: 5 minutes

Ingredients:

- 1 ripe avocado, peeled and pitted
- 1 cup fresh spinach leaves
- 1 cup unsweet almond milk (or any non-dairy milk)
- 1 tablespoon honey (optional)
- Ice cubes (optional)

Directions:

1. In a blender, combine the avocado, spinach, almond milk, and honey (if using).
2. Blend until smooth and creamy.
3. Put ice cubes if desired for a colder texture.
4. Pour into glasses and serve immediately.

Nutrition Information (per serving):

Calories: 180, Total Fat: 14g, Carbohydrates: 14g, Fiber: 7g, Protein: 3g

Strawberry Kiwi Delight

Servings: 1-2

Prep Time: 7 minutes

Ingredients:

- 1 cup fresh strawberries, hulled
- 2 ripe kiwis, peeled and sliced
- ½ cup plain Greek yogurt (low-fat or non-fat)
- ½ cup cold water or coconut water
- 1 teaspoon honey (optional)

Directions:

1. Combine the strawberries, kiwis, Greek yogurt, cold water, and honey (if using) in a blender.
2. Blend until smooth.

3. Taste and put more honey if desired for sweetness.
4. Pour into glasses and serve chilled.

Calories: 120, Total Fat: 1g, Carbohydrates: 24g, Fiber: 5g, Protein: 5g

Cucumber Mint Cooler

Servings: 1-2

Prep Time: 5 minutes

Ingredients:

- 1 large cucumber, peeled and chopped
- ½ cup fresh mint leaves
- Juice of 1 lime
- 1-2 teaspoons honey (optional)
- 1 cup cold water or coconut water
- Ice cubes (optional)

Directions:

1. In a blender, combine the cucumber, mint leaves, lime juice, honey (if using), and cold water.
2. Blend until smooth.
3. Taste and balance sweetness with more honey if needed.
4. Add ice cubes for a cooler temperature, if desired.
5. Spread into glasses and garnish with mint leaves. Serve immediately.

Nutrition Information (per serving):

Calories: 45, Total Fat: 0.5g, Carbohydrates: 11g, Fiber: 2g, Protein: 1g

Blueberry Banana Oat Smoothie

Servings: 1-2

Prep Time: 8 minutes

Ingredients:

- 1 ripe banana
- 1 cup fresh or frozen blueberries
- ½ cup rolled oats (gluten-free if necessary)
- 1 cup unsweet almond milk (or any non-dairy milk)
- 1 tablespoon chia seeds (optional)

Directions:

1. Combine the banana, blueberries, rolled oats, almond milk, and chia seeds (if applying) in a blender.
2. Blend until smooth and creamy.
3. Pour into glasses and serve immediately.

Nutrition Information (per serving):

Calories: 230, Total Fat: 4g, Carbohydrates: 45g, Fiber: 9g, Protein: 6g

Cherry Vanilla Smoothie

Servings: 1-2

Prep Time: 6 minutes

Ingredients:

- 1 cup frozen cherries, pitted
- ½ cup plain Greek yogurt (low-fat or non-fat)
- 1 teaspoon pure vanilla extract
- 1 cup almond milk (or any non-dairy milk)
- 1 tablespoon honey (optional)

Directions:

1. In a blender, combine the frozen cherries, Greek yogurt, vanilla extract, almond milk, and honey (if using).
2. Blend until smooth.
3. Taste and balance sweetness with more honey if desired.
4. Pour into glasses and serve immediately.

Nutrition Information (per serving):

Calories: 160, Total Fat: 2g, Carbohydrates: 32g, Fiber: 4g, Protein: 7g

Pineapple Coconut Smoothie

Serving: 1-2

Prep Time: 5 minutes

Cook Time: 0 minutes

Ingredients:

- 1 cup frozen pineapple chunks
- 1/2 cup coconut milk (unsweetened)
- 1/2 cup plain Greek yogurt (low-fat)
- 1 tablespoon honey (optional for sweetness)
- Ice cubes (optional)

Directions:

1. In a blender, combine frozen pineapple chunks, coconut milk, Greek yogurt, and honey (if using).
2. Mix them on high speed until the mixture is smooth and creamy.
3. If preferred, add a few ice cubes and blend again for a cooler consistency.
4. Pour into a glass and serve immediately.

Nutrition Information (per serving):

Calories: Approx. 180-200, Total Fat: 8-10g, Carbohydrates: 20-25g, Protein: 8-10g

Mango Ginger Smoothie

Serving: 1-2

Prep Time: 5 minutes

Cook Time: 0 minutes

Ingredients:

- 1 cup frozen mango chunks
- 1/2 cup plain yogurt (low-fat)
- 1/2 cup almond milk (unsweetened)
- 1 teaspoon grated ginger
- 1 tablespoon honey (optional for sweetness)
- Ice cubes (optional)

Directions:

1. Place frozen mango chunks, yogurt, almond milk, grated ginger, and honey (if using) into a blender.
2. Mix until the mixture is smooth and all ingredients are well combined.
3. Add ice cubes if a colder texture is desired, then blend again briefly.
4. Pour into a glass and serve immediately.

Nutrition Information (per serving):

Calories: Approx. 150-180, Total Fat: 4-6g, Carbohydrates: 25-30g, Protein: 6-8g

Peanut Butter Banana Smoothie

Serving: 1-2

Prep Time: 5 minutes

Cook Time: 0 minutes

Ingredients:

- 1 ripe banana
- 2 tablespoons natural peanut butter
- 1 cup almond milk (unsweetened)
- 1/2 cup plain Greek yogurt (low-fat)
- Ice cubes (optional)

Directions:

1. Peel and slice the banana.
2. In a blender, combine banana slices, peanut butter, almond milk, and Greek yogurt.
3. Combine until the compound is smooth and creamy.
4. Add ice cubes if preferred and blend again briefly.
5. Pour into a glass and serve immediately.

Nutrition Information (per serving):

Calories: Approx. 250-280, Total Fat: 14-16g, Carbohydrates: 20-25g, Protein: 10-12g

Raspberry Spinach Smoothie

Serving: 1-2

Prep Time: 5 minutes

Cook Time: 0 minutes

Ingredients:

- 1 cup fresh or frozen raspberries
- 1 cup fresh spinach leaves
- 1/2 cup plain yogurt (low-fat)
- 1/2 cup almond milk (unsweetened)
- 1 tablespoon honey (optional for sweetness)
- Ice cubes (optional)

Directions:

1. In a blender, combine raspberries, fresh spinach leaves, yogurt, almond milk, and honey (if using).
2. Meld until all ingredients are thoroughly mixed and the mixture is smooth.
3. Add ice cubes if desired and blend briefly for a cooler drink.
4. Pour into a glass and serve immediately.

Nutrition Information (per serving):

Calories: Approx. 120-150, Total Fat: 3-5g, Carbohydrates: 20-25g, Protein: 5-7g

Carrot Orange Smoothie

Serving: 1-2

Prep Time: 5 minutes

Cook Time: 0 minutes

Ingredients:

- 1 large carrot, peeled and chopped
- 1 large orange, peeled and segmented
- 1/2 cup plain Greek yogurt (low-fat)
- 1/2 cup almond milk (unsweetened)
- 1 tablespoon honey (optional for sweetness)
- Ice cubes (optional)

Directions:

1. Place chopped carrot, segmented orange, Greek yogurt, almond milk, and honey (if using) into a blender.
2. Combine until the mixture is smooth and all ingredients are well combined.
3. Add ice cubes for a colder texture, if desired, and blend briefly.
4. Pour into a glass and serve immediately.

Nutrition Information (per serving):

Calories: Approx. 130-160, Total Fat: 3-4g, Carbohydrates: 20-25g, Protein: 7-9g

Apple Cinnamon Smoothie

Serving: 1-2

Prep Time: 5 minutes

Ingredients:

- 1 medium-sized apple, peeled and chopped
- 1/2 cup plain yogurt (low-fat or dairy-free alternative)
- 1/2 teaspoon ground cinnamon
- 1 tablespoon honey (optional)
- 1/2 cup almond milk (unsweetened)

Directions:

1. Place the chopped apple, yogurt, cinnamon, honey (if using), and almond milk in a blender.
2. Blend until smooth and creamy.
3. Serve immediately and enjoy!

Nutrition Information (per serving):

Calories: Approx. 150, Fat: 3g, Carbohydrates: 30g, Fiber: 5g, Protein: 4g

Turmeric Mango Smoothie

Serving: 1-2

Prep Time: 5 minutes

Ingredients:

- 1 ripe mango, peeled and diced
- 1/2 teaspoon ground turmeric
- 1/2 cup coconut water
- 1/2 cup Greek yogurt (low-fat or dairy-free alternative)
- 1 tablespoon chia seeds (optional)

Directions:

1. Combine the diced mango, ground turmeric, coconut water, Greek yogurt, and chia seeds (if using) in a blender.
2. Blend until smooth and creamy.
3. Pour into glasses and serve chilled.

Nutrition Information (per serving):

Calories: Approx. 180, Fat: 4g, Carbohydrates: 30g, Fiber: 5g, Protein: 8g

Grapefruit Berry Smoothie

Serving: 1-2

Prep Time: 5 minutes

Ingredients:

- 1/2 grapefruit, peeled and deseeded
- 1 cup mixed berries (strawberries, blueberries, raspberries)
- 1/2 cup coconut milk (unsweetened)
- 1 tablespoon honey or maple syrup (optional)

Directions:

1. Place the grapefruit segments, mixed berries, coconut milk, and honey or maple syrup (if applying) in a blender.
2. Blend until smooth and well combined.
3. Pour into glasses and serve immediately.

Nutrition Information (per serving):

Calories: Approx. 140, Fat: 5g, Carbohydrates: 25g, Fiber: 7g, Protein: 2g

Watermelon Mint Smoothie

Serving: 1-2

Prep Time: 5 minutes

Ingredients:

- 2 cups seedless watermelon, cubed
- 5-6 fresh mint leaves
- 1/2 cup plain Greek yogurt (low-fat or dairy-free alternative)
- 1 tablespoon lime juice
- 1-2 teaspoons honey (optional)

Directions:

1. Combine the watermelon cubes, fresh mint leaves, Greek yogurt, lime juice, and honey (if using) in a blender.
2. Blend until smooth and thoroughly mixed.
3. Serve immediately over ice, if desired.

Nutrition Information (per serving):

Calories: Approx. 100, Fat: 1g, Carbohydrates: 20g, Fiber: 1g, Protein: 5g

Serving: 1-2

Prep Time: 5 minutes

Ingredients:

- 1 cup mixed berries (strawberries, blueberries, raspberries)
- 1/2 ripe banana
- 1/2 cup coconut milk (unsweetened)
- 1/4 cup basic Greek yogurt (low-fat or dairy-free alternative)

Directions:

1. Place the mixed berries, ripe banana, coconut milk, and Greek yogurt in a blender.
2. Blend until smooth and creamy.
3. Serve immediately for best taste.

Nutrition Information (per serving):

Calories: Approx. 160, Fat: 6g, Carbohydrates: 25g, Fiber: 6g, Protein: 5g

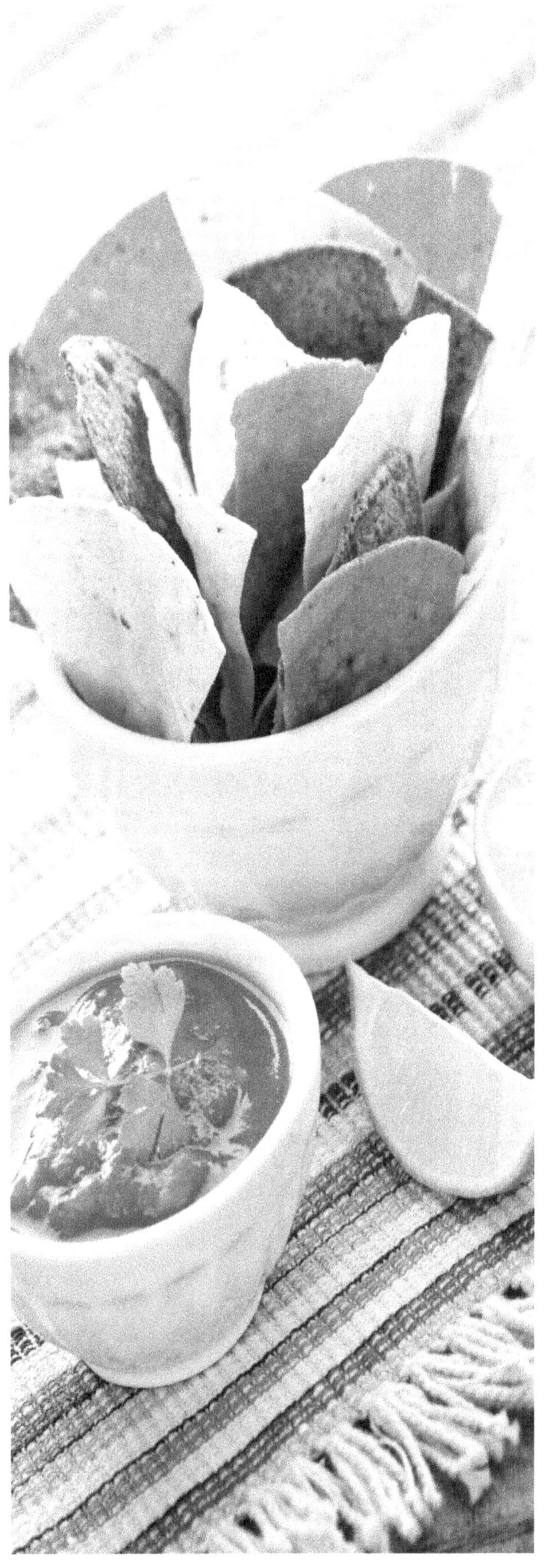

Fruit Salad

Serving: 1-2

Prep Time: 10 minutes

Ingredients:

- 1 cup mixed fruits (such as diced apples, bananas, grapes, and berries)
- 1 tablespoon honey (optional)
- Fresh lemon juice (from 1 lemon)

Directions:

1. Wash and prepare the fruits. Cut them into bite-sized pieces.
2. In a mixing bowl, combine the fruits.
3. Squeeze fresh lemon juice over the fruits to prevent browning.
4. Optionally, drizzle honey over the fruits for sweetness.
5. Gently toss the fruits to coat evenly.
6. Serve immediately or chill before serving.

Nutrition Information (per serving):

Calories: Varies based on fruit selection, Total Fat: Varies, Carbohydrates: Varies, Protein: Varies, Fiber: Varies

Vegetable Sticks with Hummus

Serving: 1-2

Prep Time: 15 minutes

Ingredients:

- Assorted fresh vegetables (carrots, celery, bell peppers, cucumber, etc.), cut into sticks
- ½ cup hummus

Directions:

1. Wash and cut the vegetables into stick shapes.
2. Arrange the vegetable sticks on a plate.
3. Serve with a side of hummus for dipping.

Nutrition Information (per serving):

Calories: Varies based on vegetables and hummus, Total Fat: Varies, Carbohydrates: Varies, Protein: Varies, Fiber: Varies

Greek Yogurt with Berries

Serving: 1-2

Prep Time: 5 minutes

Ingredients:

- 1 cup Greek yogurt
- ½ cup assorted berries (such as strawberries, blueberries, raspberries)

Directions:

- Scoop Greek yogurt into serving bowls.
- Wash and add the mixed berries on top of the yogurt.
- Serve chilled.

Nutrition Information (per serving):

Calories: Varies based on yogurt and berries, Total Fat: Varies, Carbohydrates: Varies, Protein: Varies, Fiber: Varies

Rice Cakes with Almond Butter

Serving: 1-2

Prep Time: 5 minutes

Ingredients:

- 2 rice cakes
- 2 tablespoons almond butter (unsweetened)

Directions:

1. Spread almond butter evenly over each rice cake.
2. Serve immediately.

Nutrition Information (per serving):

Calories: Varies based on rice cakes and almond butter, Total Fat: Varies, Carbohydrates: Varies, Protein: Varies, Fiber: Varies

Baked Apple Chips

Serving: 1-2

Prep Time: 10 minutes

Cook Time: 1 hour

Ingredients:

- 2 apples
- Cinnamon (optional)

Directions:

1. Set out the oven to 200°F (95°C).
2. Wash and thinly slice the apples.
3. Lay the apple chunks on a baking sheet lined with parchment paper.
4. Optionally, sprinkle cinnamon over the apple slices for added flavor.
5. Bake for about 1 hour or until the apples turn crisp, flipping them halfway through.
6. Let the apple chips cool before serving.

Nutrition Information (per serving):

Calories: Varies based on apple size and quantity, Total Fat: Varies, Carbohydrates: Varies, Protein: Varies, Fiber: Varies

Cottage Cheese with Pineapple

Servings: 1-2

Prep Time: 5 minutes

Ingredients:

- 1 cup cottage cheese (low-fat)
- ½ cup pineapple strips (fresh or canned in juice)

Directions:

1. In a bowl, place the cottage cheese.
2. Add the pineapple chunks on top.
3. Gently mix together.
4. Serve immediately.

Nutrition Information (per serving):

Calories: 150, Protein: 15g, Fat: 3g, Carbohydrates: 15g, Fiber: 1g

Whole Grain Crackers with Avocado

Servings: 1-2

Prep Time: 5 minutes

Ingredients:

- 4-6 whole grain crackers
- 1 ripe avocado, mashed
- Pinch of salt (optional)

Directions:

1. Spread the mashed avocado evenly on the whole grain crackers.
2. Add a pinch of salt if desired.
3. Serve immediately.

Nutrition Information (per serving):

Calories: 180, Protein: 4g, Fat: 10g, Carbohydrates: 20g, Fiber: 6g

Homemade Trail Mix

Servings: 4

Prep Time: 5 minutes

Ingredients:

- 1 cup mixed unsalted nuts (almonds, walnuts, cashews)
- ½ cup dried cranberries
- ½ cup pumpkin seeds

Directions:

1. Mix all ingredients in a bowl.
2. Store in an airtight container.

Calories: 200, Protein: 6g, Fat: 15g, Carbohydrates: 12g, Fiber: 3g

Popcorn

Servings: 2

Prep Time: 5 minutes

Cook Time: 5 minutes

Ingredients:

- ½ cup popcorn kernels
- 2 tablespoons olive oil
- Salt to taste (optional)

Directions:

1. Gush the olive oil in a large pot over medium heat.
2. Add the popcorn kernels, cover with a lid, and shake occasionally.
3. Once popping slows down, remove from heat.
4. Add salt if desired.
5. Serve immediately.

Nutrition Information (per serving):

Calories: 120, Protein: 3g, Fat: 8g, Carbohydrates: 10g, Fiber: 2g

Fruit Smoothie

Servings: 1-2

Prep Time: 5 minutes

Ingredients:

- 1 cup mixed frozen berries (strawberries, blueberries, raspberries)
- 1 ripe banana
- 1 cup unsweetened almond milk or water
- 1 tablespoon honey (optional)

Directions:

1. In a blender, combine all ingredients.
2. Blend until smooth.
3. Add honey if desired for sweetness.
4. Serve immediately.

Nutrition Information (per serving):

Calories: 150, Protein: 3g, Fat: 1g, Carbohydrates: 35g, Fiber: 6g

Vegetable Chips

Serving: 1-2

Prep Time: 10 minutes

Cook Time: 20-25 minutes

Ingredients:

- Assorted vegetables (sweet potatoes, zucchini, beets, etc.)
- Olive oil
- Salt and pepper to taste

Directions:

1. Preheat oven to 350°F (175°C).
2. Wash and slice vegetables thinly using a mandoline slicer or a sharp knife.
3. Place sliced vegetables in a bowl, dribble with olive oil, and dribble with salt and pepper. Toss to coat evenly.
4. Arrange the slices in a single layer on a baking sheet lined with parchment paper.
5. Bake for 20-25 minutes or until the edges turn golden brown and the chips are crisp.
6. Let cool before serving.

Nutrition Information: (per serving)

Calories: Varies, Fat: Varies, Carbohydrates: Varies, Fiber: Varies, Protein: Varies

Chia Seed Pudding

Serving: 1-2

Prep Time: 5 minutes

Chilling Time: 2 hours or overnight

Ingredients:

- 1/4 cup chia seeds
- 1 cup sour soy milk or coconut milk
- 1 teaspoon honey or maple syrup (optional)
- Fresh fruits for topping (e.g., berries, sliced banana)

Directions:

1. In a bowl, mix chia seeds, almond/coconut milk, and sweetener (if using). Stir well.
2. Cover the bowl and refrigerate for at least 2 hours or overnight, allowing the chia seeds to soak the liquid and form a pudding-like consistency.
3. Before serving, stir the mixture again. Add fresh fruits on top if desired.

Nutrition Information: (per serving)

Calories: Approximately 150, Fat: 8g, Carbohydrates: 15g, Fiber: 10g, Protein: 5g

Hummus Cucumber Bites

Serving: 1-2

Prep Time: 10 minutes

Ingredients:

- Cucumber, sliced into rounds
- Hummus
- Paprika (optional, for garnish)

Directions:

1. Dice up the cucumber into rounds about 1/4 inch thick.
2. Spoon a small dollop of hummus onto each cucumber slice.
3. Sprinkle paprika for added flavor if desired.
4. Arrange on a plate and serve immediately.

Nutrition Information: (per serving)

Calories: Approximately 50-60, Fat: 2g, Carbohydrates: 6g, Fiber: 2g, Protein: 2g

Frozen Grapes

Serving: 1-2

Prep Time: 5 minutes

Freezing Time: 2 hours

Ingredients:

- Fresh grapes (seedless)

Directions:

1. Wash and pat dry the grapes.
2. Settle the grapes in a single layer on a baking sheet or plate.
3. Freeze for at least 2 hours or until solid.
4. Serve the frozen grapes directly as a refreshing snack.

Nutrition Information: (per serving)

Calories: Approximately 60-70, Fat: 0g, Carbohydrates: 15-20g, Fiber: 1-2g, Protein: 1g

Baked Tortilla Chips with Salsa

Serving: 1-2

Prep Time: 10 minutes

Cook Time: 10-12 minutes

Ingredients:

- Corn tortillas
- Olive oil spray
- Salt

- Salsa (store-bought or homemade)

Directions:

1. Preheat oven to 350°F (175°C).
2. Cut the tortillas into wedges or desired shapes.
3. Arrange the tortilla pieces on a baking sheet lined with parchment paper.
4. Dribble with olive oil and dust with salt.
5. Bake for 10-12 minutes or until the chips are crisp and lightly golden.
6. Serve with salsa on the side for dipping.

Nutrition Information: (per serving, without salsa)

Calories: Approximately 80-100, Fat: 1-2g, Carbohydrates: 15-20g, Fiber: 2-3g, Protein: 2g

Apple Slices with Almond Butter

Servings: 1-2

Prep Time: 5 minutes

Ingredients:

- 1 apple, sliced
- 2 tablespoons almond butter

Directions:

1. Wash the apple thoroughly and slice it into thin pieces.
2. Take almond butter and spread it on the apple slices.
3. Fix the slices on a plate and serve.

Nutrition Information (per serving):

Calories: Approximately 150 kcal, Fat: 9g, Carbohydrates: 18g, Protein: 3g

Low-Fat Yogurt Parfait

Servings: 1-2

Prep Time: 5 minutes

Ingredients:

- 1 cup low-fat yogurt
- 1/2 cup granola
- 1/2 cup fresh berries (blueberries, strawberries, raspberries)

Directions:

1. Take a serving glass or bowl.
2. Layer the yogurt, granola, and fresh berries alternatively.
3. Redo the layers until the glass or bowl is filled.
4. Serve immediately.

Nutrition Information (per serving):

Calories: Approximately 250 kcal, Fat: 5g, Carbohydrates: 40g, Protein: 10g

Celery and Peanut Butter

Servings: 1-2

Prep Time: 5 minutes

Ingredients:

- 4-5 celery stalks, washed and trimmed
- 2 tablespoons peanut butter (low-fat)

Directions:

1. Spread peanut butter along the hollow side of the celery stalks.
2. Place them on a plate and serve.

Nutrition Information (per serving):

Calories: Approximately 120 kcal, Fat: 8g, Carbohydrates: 8g, Protein: 4g

Roasted Chickpeas

Servings: 1-2

Prep Time: 5 minutes

Cook Time: 30 minutes

Ingredients:

- 1 can (15 oz) chickpeas, drained off and rinsed
- 1 tablespoon olive oil
- Seasonings (such as paprika, garlic powder, salt) to taste

Directions:

1. Set out the oven to 400°F (200°C).
2. Pat dry the chickpeas using a paper towel.
3. Into a bowl, toss chickpeas with olive oil and seasonings.
4. Roll out the chickpeas on a baking sheet lined with parchment paper.
5. Cook into the oven for 30 minutes, stirring halfway through.
6. Let them cool before serving.

Nutrition Information (per serving):

Calories: Approximately 200 kcal, Fat: 7g, Carbohydrates: 28g, Protein: 8g

Fruit Skewers

Servings: 1-2

Prep Time: 10 minutes

Ingredients:

- Assorted fruits (such as strawberries, pineapple chunks, grapes, melon balls)

Directions:

1. Wash and prepare the fruits, cutting them into bite-sized pieces if needed.
2. Thread the fruit pieces onto skewers in any pattern you prefer.
3. Arrange on a plate and serve.

Nutrition Information (per serving):

Calories: Varies, Fat: Varies, Carbohydrates: Varies, Protein: Varies

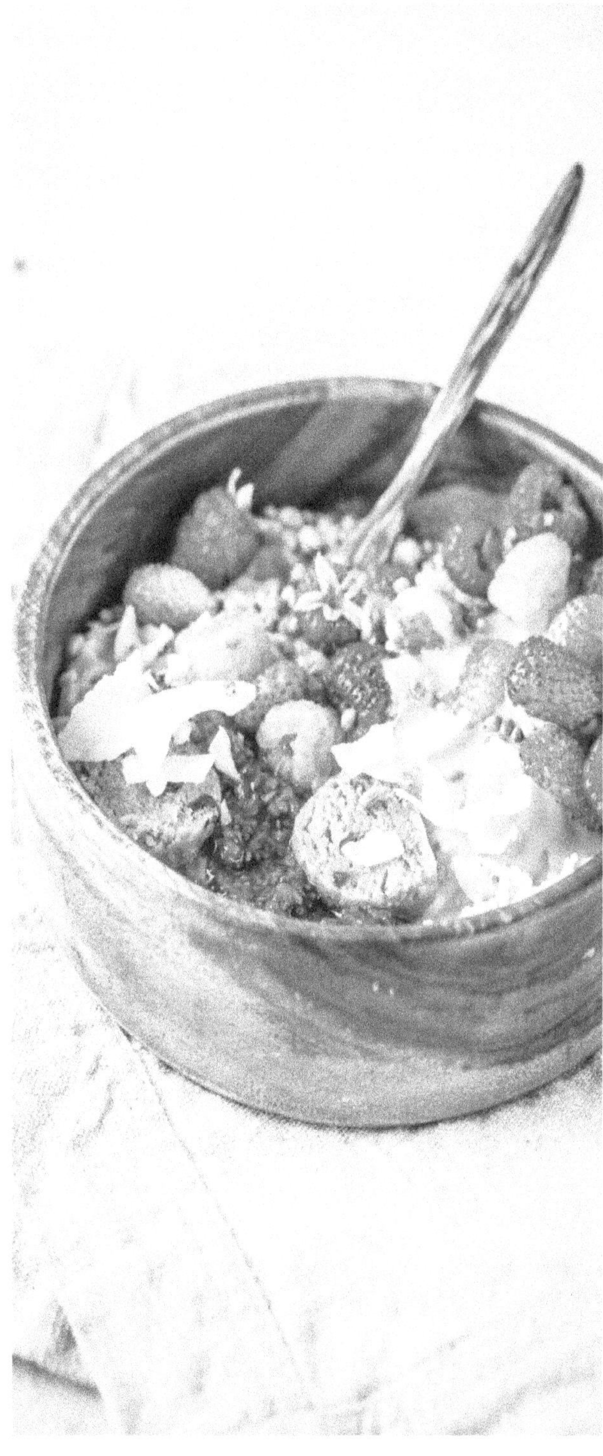

Homemade Vegetable Broth

Servings: 4-6

Prep Time: 10 minutes

Cook Time: 1 hour

Ingredients:

- 2 large carrots, chopped
- 2 celery stalks, chopped
- 1 onion, peeled and quartered
- 2 garlic cloves, crushed
- 1 potato, diced
- 6 cups water
- 1 teaspoon dried thyme
- 1 teaspoon dried parsley
- Salt to taste (optional)

Directions:

1. In a large pot, combine all the vegetables and water.
2. Add dried thyme and parsley. Bring the mixture to a boil.
3. Decrease the heat, cover, and let it simmer for about 1 hour.
4. Once done, strain the broth through a fine-mesh sieve or cheesecloth.
5. Discard the vegetables and season with salt if desired.
6. Allow it to cool before storing in the refrigerator for up to 3-4 days.

Nutrition Information (per serving):

Calories: 15, Carbohydrates: 3g, Fiber: 1g, Protein: 0.5g, Fat: 0g

Cooked Quinoa

Servings: 2-3

Prep Time: 5 minutes

Cook Time: 15-20 minutes

Ingredients:

- 1 cup quinoa, rinsed
- 2 cups water or low-sodium vegetable broth

Directions:

1. Rinse quinoa thoroughly in a fine-mesh strainer.
2. In a pot, bring water or vegetable broth to a boil.
3. Add quinoa, reduce heat, cover, and simmer down for 15-20 minutes or until the liquid is absorbed.
4. Stuff quinoa with a fork and let it sit for a few minutes before serving.

Nutrition Information (per serving):

Calories: 111, Carbohydrates: 19g, Fiber: 2.6g, Protein: 4g, Fat: 1.8g

Brown Rice

Servings: 2-3

Prep Time: 5 minutes

Cook Time: 45-50 minutes

Ingredients:

- 1 cup brown rice
- 2 cups water

Directions:

1. Rinse brown rice in a fine-mesh strainer until water runs clear.
2. Take a pot, bring water to a boil.
3. Add up rice, reduce heat, cover, and simmer for 45-50 minutes or until tender and water is absorbed.
4. Let it sit covered for a few minutes before serving.

Nutrition Information (per serving):

Calories: 108, Carbohydrates: 22.4g, Fiber: 1.8g, Protein: 2.3g, Fat: 0.9g

Steamed Vegetables

Servings: 2

Prep Time: 10 minutes

Cook Time: 5-10 minutes

Ingredients:

- Assorted vegetables (broccoli, carrots, zucchini, bell peppers, etc.), washed and chopped

Directions:

1. Place a steamer basket in a pot with a small amount of water.
2. Add chopped vegetables to the basket.
3. Cover and steam for 5-10 minutes or until vegetables are tender but still slightly crisp.
4. Season with herbs or a sprinkle of lemon juice if desired before serving.

Nutrition Information (per serving):

Depends on the vegetables used; generally low in calories and rich in vitamins and fiber.

Boiled Potatoes

Servings: 2-3

Prep Time: 10 minutes

Cook Time: 20-25 minutes

Ingredients:

- 3-4 medium-sized potatoes, washed and diced

Directions:

1. Put the diced potatoes in a pot and cover with water.
2. After a boil and reduce heat to a simmer.
3. Heat it for 20-25 minutes or until potatoes are tender when pierced with a fork.
4. Drain and serve.

Nutrition Information (per serving):

Calories: 145, Carbohydrates: 33.6g, Fiber: 3.6g, Protein: 3.6g, Fat: 0.2g

Cooked Lentils

Serving: 2 servings

Prep Time: 5 minutes

Cook Time: 20-25 minutes

Ingredients:

- 1 cup dried lentils
- 2 cups water or low-sodium vegetable broth
- 1 teaspoon olive oil (optional)
- Salt and pepper to taste

Directions:

1. Rinse lentils under cold water and drain.
2. In a pot, combine lentils and water or broth. Boil it.
3. Remove the heat to low, cover, and simmer down for 20-25 minutes until lentils are tender but not mushy.
4. If desired, stir in olive oil and season with salt and pepper.
5. Serve as a side dish or as a base for other meals.

Nutrition Information (per serving):

Calories: 220, Protein: 18g, Carbohydrates: 38g, Fat: 1g, Fiber: 16g

Oatmeal

Serving: 1 serving

Prep Time: 2 minutes

Cook Time: 5 minutes

Ingredients:

- 1/2 cup rolled oats
- 1 cup water or low-fat milk
- 1 tablespoon honey or maple syrup (optional)
- Cinnamon or nutmeg (optional)

Directions:

1. Take a small saucepan, bring water or milk to a boil.
2. Stir in the rolled oats up and reduce heat to medium-low.
3. Roast it for 5 minutes, stirring occasionally until oats are soft and creamy.
4. Sweeten up with honey or maple syrup if desired. Put a pinch of cinnamon or nutmeg for flavor.
5. Remove from heat and let it sit for a minute before serving.

Nutrition Information (per serving):

Calories: 150, Protein: 5g, Carbohydrates: 27g, Fat: 2.5g, Fiber: 4g

Whole Grain Pasta

Serving: 2 servings

Prep Time: 2 minutes

Cook Time: 10-12 minutes

Ingredients:

- 1 cup whole grain pasta (such as whole wheat or brown rice pasta)
- Water
- Salt (optional)

Directions:

1. Take a pot of water to a boil.
2. Add up the pasta and cook according to package instructions until al dente (usually 10-12 minutes).
3. Drain off the pasta and rinse it under cold water to stop the cooking process.
4. Season lightly with salt if desired.
5. Serve with your choice of toppings or sauce (like the herb-infused tomato sauce).

Nutrition Information (per serving):

Calories: 200, Protein: 7g, Carbohydrates: 40g, Fat: 1.5g, Fiber: 6g

Low-Fat Vinaigrette

Serving: Makes about 1/2 cup

Prep Time: 5 minutes

Ingredients:

- 3 tablespoons extra virgin olive oil
- 2 tablespoons vinegar (such as apple cider or red wine vinegar)
- 1 teaspoon Dijon mustard
- 1/2 teaspoon honey or maple syrup
- Salt and pepper to taste

Directions:

1. Take a small bowl, combine it together olive oil, vinegar, mustard, and honey or maple syrup.
2. Season with salt and pepper to taste.
3. Adjust ingredients to achieve desired taste and consistency.
4. Keep it in a sealed container in the refrigerator for up to a week.

Nutrition Information (per tablespoon):

Calories: 50, Protein: 0g, Carbohydrates: 1g, Fat: 5g, Fiber: 0g

Herb-Infused Tomato Sauce

Serving: 4 servings

Prep Time: 5 minutes

Cook Time: 20-25 minutes

Ingredients:

- 1 can (14 oz) low-sodium crushed tomatoes
- 2 cloves garlic, minced
- 1 tablespoon extra-virgin olive oil
- 1 teaspoon dried basil
- 1 teaspoon dried oregano
- Salt and pepper to taste

Directions:

1. Sprinkle olive oil in a saucepan over medium heat.
2. Add minced garlic and sauté for 1-2 minutes until fragrant but not browned.
3. Pour in the crushed tomatoes and add basil and oregano.
4. Season with salt and pepper.
5. Simmer down for 20-25 minutes, stirring at times, until the sauce thickens.
6. Adjust seasoning to taste.
7. Use as a topping for whole grain pasta or as desired.

Nutrition Information (per serving):

Calories: 50, Protein: 1g, Carbohydrates: 6g, Fat: 3g, Fiber: 2g

Lemon Herb Dressing

Servings: 2

Prep Time: 5 minutes

Ingredients:

- 2 tablespoons fresh lemon juice
- 1 tablespoon extra-virgin olive oil
- 1 teaspoon finely diced fresh herbs (such as basil, parsley, or dill)
- Pinch of salt and pepper

Directions:

1. Into a small bowl, whisk together the lemon juice, olive oil, chopped herbs, salt, and pepper.
2. Taste and adjust seasoning if needed.
3. Serve immediately over a salad or refrigerate in a sealed case for up to 3 days.

Nutrition Information: (per serving)

Calories: 60, Total Fat: 7g, Carbohydrates: 1g, Protein: 0g, Fiber: 0g, Sodium: 150mg

Greek Yogurt Ranch Dip

Servings: 2

Prep Time: 5 minutes

Ingredients:

- ½ cup plain Greek yogurt (low-fat or fat-free)
- 1 tablespoon chopped fresh chives
- 1 teaspoon dried dill
- ½ teaspoon garlic powder
- Salt and pepper to taste

Directions:

1. Take a mixing bowl, combine the Greek yogurt, chives, dill, garlic powder, salt, and pepper.
2. Whisk them well until all ingredients are thoroughly combined.
3. Refrigerate for at least 30 minutes before serving to enhance flavors.

Nutrition Information: (per serving)

Calories: 40, Total Fat: 0g, Carbohydrates: 3g, Protein: 7g, Fiber: 0g, Sodium: 40mg

Servings: 2

Prep Time: 2 minutes

Cook Time: 10 minutes

Ingredients:

- ½ cup balsamic vinegar
- 1 tablespoon honey (optional)

Directions:

1. Take a small sauce pan, bring the balsamic vinegar to a gentle boil over medium heat.
2. Decrease heat and simmer, stirring occasionally, until the vinegar is reduced by half and thickened (about 8-10 minutes). Optionally, add honey for sweetness if desired.
3. Allow the glaze to cool before using or keeping in an airtight jar in the refrigerator for up to a week.

Nutrition Information: (per serving)

Calories: 50, Total Fat: 0g, Carbohydrates: 12g, Protein: 0g, Fiber: 0g, Sodium: 10mg

Tahini Sauce

Servings: 2

Prep Time: 5 minutes

Ingredients:

- 2 tablespoons tahini
- 2 tablespoons water
- 1 tablespoon lemon juice
- 1 small garlic clove, minced
- Pinch of salt

Directions:

1. Take a small bowl, whisk together tahini, water, lemon juice, ground garlic, and salt until smooth and well combined.
2. Adjust consistency by adding more water if needed.
3. Set out immediately or store in the refrigerator in an airtight jar for up to 5 days.

Nutrition Information: (per serving)

Calories: 80, Total Fat: 7g, Carbohydrates: 3g, Protein: 2g, Fiber: 1g, Sodium: 75mg

Apple Cider Vinegar Dressing

Servings: 2

Prep Time: 5 minutes

Ingredients:

- 2 tablespoons apple cider vinegar
- 2 tablespoons extra-virgin olive oil
- 1 teaspoon Dijon mustard
- 1 teaspoon honey
- Pinch of salt and pepper

Directions:

1. Take a small bowl, whisk together apple cider vinegar, olive oil, Dijon mustard, honey, salt, and pepper until emulsified.
2. Taste and adjust seasoning according to preference.
3. Use immediately or store in the refrigerator for up to a week in an airtight container.

Nutrition Information: (per serving)

Calories: 120, Total Fat: 14g, Carbohydrates: 2g, Protein: 0g, Fiber: 0g, Sodium: 80mg

Soy Ginger Sauce

Servings: 2-4

Prep Time: 5 minutes

Cook Time: 5 minutes

Ingredients:

- 1/4 cup low-sodium soy sauce
- 1 tablespoon grated ginger
- 1 tablespoon rice vinegar
- 1 teaspoon honey
- 1 clove garlic, minced
- 1 teaspoon sesame oil (optional)

1. Take a small bowl, whisk together soy sauce, grated ginger, rice vinegar, honey, minced garlic, and sesame oil (if using).
2. Set the mixture in a small saucepan over low heat for 5 minutes, stirring occasionally.
3. Remove from heat and let it cool before serving.
4. Use as a dipping sauce or to flavor stir-fried vegetables or lean protein.

Nutrition Information (per serving):

Calories: 25, Total Fat: 0.5g, Sodium: 670mg, Total Carbohydrates: 4g, Protein: 2g

Avocado Lime Dressing

Servings: 2-4

Prep Time: 10 minutes

Cook Time: 0 minutes

Ingredients:

- 1 ripe avocado, peeled and pitted
- Juice of 1 lime
- 2 tablespoons olive oil
- 1 tablespoon chopped fresh cilantro
- Salt and pepper to taste

Directions:

1. Take a blender or food processor, combine the avocado, lime juice, olive oil, and cilantro. Blend until smooth.
2. Season with salt and pepper to taste.
3. Let it cool for 30 minutes before serving to allow flavors to meld.
4. Drizzle over salads or use as a dip for vegetables.

Nutrition Information (per serving):

Calories: 90, Total Fat: 9g, Sodium: 5mg, Total Carbohydrates: 3g, Protein: 1g

Mango Salsa

Servings: 2-4

Prep Time: 15 minutes

Cook Time: 0 minutes

Ingredients:

- 1 ripe mango, diced
- 1/2 red bell pepper, diced
- 1/4 cup diced red onion
- 1 tablespoon chopped fresh cilantro
- Juice of 1 lime
- Salt and pepper to taste

Directions:

1. In a bowl, combine diced mango, red bell pepper, red onion, cilantro, and lime juice. Mix well.
2. Season with salt and pepper to taste.
3. Refrigerate for 15-20 minutes before serving to enhance flavors.
4. Set out as a topping for grilled chicken or fish, or as a refreshing side dish.

Nutrition Information (per serving):

Calories: 45, Total Fat: 0.5g, Sodium: 2mg, Total Carbohydrates: 11g, Protein: 1g

Hummus

Servings: 4-6

Prep Time: 10 minutes

Cook Time: 0 minutes

Ingredients:

- 1 can (15 ounces) low-sodium chickpeas, drained and rinsed
- 2 tablespoons tahini
- 2 tablespoons olive oil
- Juice of 1 lemon
- 1 clove garlic, minced
- 1/2 teaspoon ground cumin
- Salt to taste
- 2-3 tablespoons water (optional, for desired consistency)

Directions:

1. Take a food processor, combine chickpeas, tahini, olive oil, lemon juice, minced garlic, cumin, and a pinch of salt.
2. Blend until smooth. If needed, add water gradually to achieve the desired consistency.
3. Taste and adjust seasoning as desired.
4. Set out as a dip with raw vegetables or whole-grain crackers.

Nutrition Information (per serving):

Calories: 140, Total Fat: 8g, Sodium: 10mg, Total Carbohydrates: 15g, Protein: 5g

Low-Fat Pesto

Servings: 2-4

Prep Time: 10 minutes

Cook Time: 0 minutes

Ingredients:

- 2 cups fresh basil leaves
- 1/4 cup grated Parmesan cheese (optional)
- 1/4 cup pine nuts or walnuts
- 2 cloves garlic, minced
- 2 tablespoons olive oil
- Salt and pepper to taste

Directions:

1. Take a food processor, combine basil leaves, Parmesan cheese (if using), pine nuts or walnuts, minced garlic, olive oil, salt, and pepper.
2. Minggle until smooth, scraping down the sides as needed.
3. Taste and adjust seasoning if necessary.
4. Use as a sauce for pasta or a flavorful spread on whole-grain toast.

Nutrition Information (per serving):

Calories: 120, Total Fat: 12g, Sodium: 80mg, Total Carbohydrates: 2g, Protein: 2g

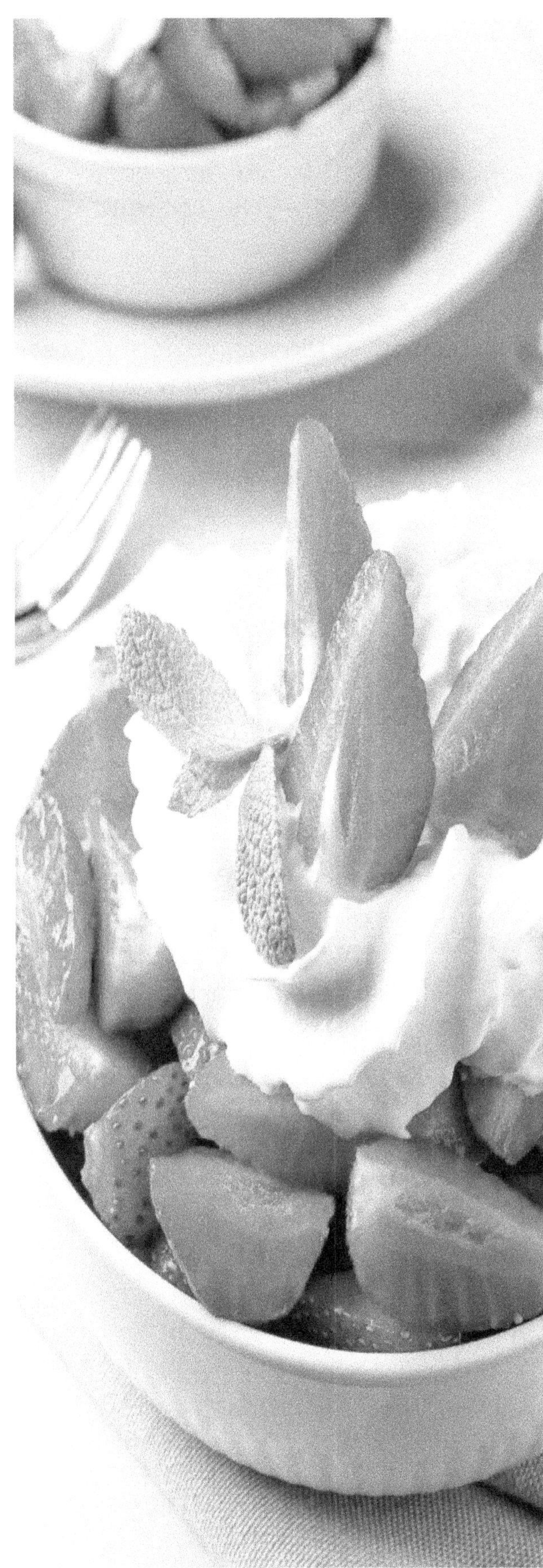

Fruit Salad with Mint

Serving: 1-2

Prep Time: 10 minutes

Ingredients:

- Assorted fruits (such as apples, grapes, berries, and melons), diced or sliced
- Fresh mint leaves, chopped

Directions:

1. Wash and prepare the fruits, cutting them into bite-sized pieces.
2. In a bowl, combine the diced fruits.
3. Sprinkle freshly chopped mint leaves over the fruit mixture.
4. Toss gently to mix.
5. Serve it straight away or refrigerate until ready to serve.

Nutrition Information (per serving):

Calories: Varies depending on fruits used, Fat: Negligible, Fiber: High, Sugar: Natural sugars from fruits

Baked Apples with Cinnamon

Serving: 1-2

Prep Time: 10 minutes

Cook Time: 30 minutes

Ingredients:

- Apples (such as Granny Smith), cored
- Ground cinnamon
- Optional: Stevia or honey (in moderation, if needed for sweetness)

Directions:

1. Preheat oven to 350°F (175°C).

2. Core the apples and place them on a baking dish.
3. Sprinkle ground cinnamon inside the cored center of each apple.
4. Optionally, drizzle a small amount of stevia or honey for sweetness (if desired).
5. Bake in the oven for about 30 minutes or until apples are tender.
6. Reduce from oven and let them cool slightly before serving.

Nutrition Information (per serving):

Calories: Varies depending on apple size, Fat: Negligible, Fiber: High, Sugar: Natural sugars from apples

Banana "Nice" Cream

Serving: 1-2

Prep Time: 5 minutes

Ingredients:

- Ripe bananas, peeled, sliced, and frozen

Directions:

1. Lay the frozen banana slices in a food processor or blender.
2. Blend until the bananas turn into a creamy consistency, resembling ice cream.
3. Serve immediately as soft-serve or freeze for a firmer texture.

Nutrition Information (per serving):

Calories: Varies depending on banana size, Fat: Negligible, Fiber: Moderate, Sugar: Natural sugars from bananas

Mixed Berry Sorbet

Serving: 1-2

Prep Time: 5 minutes

Ingredients:

- Mixed frozen berries (such as strawberries, blueberries, raspberries)
- Water
- Optional: Stevia or honey (in moderation, if needed for sweetness)

Directions:

1. Into a blender, combine the frozen berries and a splash of water.
2. Blend until smooth. If needed, add more water for preferred consistency.
3. Optionally, sweeten with a small amount of stevia or honey (if desired).
4. Serve immediately as a sorbet or freeze for a firmer texture.

Nutrition Information (per serving):

Calories: Varies depending on berry mix, Fat: Negligible, Fiber: High, Sugar: Natural sugars from berries

Frozen Yogurt Bark

Serving: 1-2

Prep Time: 10 minutes

Freezing Time: 2-3 hours

Ingredients:

- Greek yogurt (plain or flavored, low-fat or non-fat)
- Assorted toppings (such as diced fruits, nuts, seeds)

Directions:

1. Line a baking sheet with parchment paper.
2. Spread the Greek yogurt evenly onto the parchment paper.
3. Sprinkle assorted toppings over the yogurt.

4. Place in the freezer for 2-3 hours or until completely frozen.
5. Once frozen, break the yogurt bark into pieces and serve.

Nutrition Information (per serving):

Calories: Varies, Fat: Varies , Fiber: Varies, Sugar: Varies

Poached Pears

Servings: 2

Prep Time: 10 minutes

Cook Time: 20 minutes

Ingredients:

- 2 ripe pears, peeled and cored
- 2 cups water
- 1/4 cup honey or maple syrup
- 1 cinnamon stick
- 2 cloves

Directions:

1. In a saucepan, combine water, honey or maple syrup, cinnamon stick, and cloves. Bring it to a tender simmer over medium heat.
2. Add the skinned and cored pears to the simmering liquid. Cover and let them poach for about 15-20 minutes until they are tender but not too soft.
3. Once done, remove the pears from the liquid and let them cool slightly before serving. Optionally, drizzle a little of the poaching liquid over the pears for added flavor.

Nutrition Information (per serving):

Calories: 150, Total Fat: 0g, Carbohydrates: 40g, Fiber: 5g, Protein: 1g

Pumpkin Spice Muffins

Servings: 6

Prep Time: 15 minutes

Cook Time: 25 minutes

Ingredients:

- 1 cup pumpkin puree
- 2 eggs
- 1/4 cup honey or maple syrup
- 1/4 cup coconut flour
- 1 teaspoon baking powder
- 1 teaspoon pumpkin pie spice

Directions:

1. Preheat oven to 350°F (175°C). Line a muffin tin with liners.
2. In a bowl, whisk together pumpkin puree, eggs, and honey/maple syrup until well combined.
3. Add up coconut flour, baking powder, and pumpkin pie spice to the wet mixture. Mix until a smooth batter forms.
4. Carve up the batter evenly among the muffin cups.
5. Cook for 20-25 minutes or until a toothpick inserted into the muffin, comes out clean.
6. Allow the muffins to cool before serving.

Nutrition Information (per serving - 1 muffin):

Calories: 110, Total Fat: 3g, Carbohydrates: 18g, Fiber: 4g, Protein: 3g

Coconut Mango Popsicles

Servings: 4

Prep Time: 10 minutes

Freezing Time: 4 hours

Ingredients:

- 1 ripe mango, peeled and diced
- 1 cup coconut milk
- 1 tablespoon maple syrup (optional for sweetness)

Directions:

1. Place diced mango, coconut milk, and honey/maple syrup (if using) in a blender. Blend until smooth.
2. Pour the mixture into popsicle molds.
3. Insert popsicle canes and freeze for at least 4 hours or until solid.
4. To release the popsicles, run the molds under warm water for a few seconds.

Nutrition Information (per serving):

Calories: 120, Total Fat: 8g, Carbohydrates: 12g, Fiber: 1g, Protein: 1g

Baked Peaches with Yogurt

Servings: 2

Prep Time: 10 minutes

Cook Time: 15 minutes

Ingredients:

- 2 ripe peaches, halved and pitted
- 1 tablespoon honey or maple syrup
- 1/4 teaspoon cinnamon
- Greek yogurt for serving

Directions:

1. Preheat oven to 375°F (190°C).
2. Place peach halves on a baking sheet, cut side up.
3. Pour honey or maple syrup over the peaches and sprinkle with cinnamon.
4. Cook for about 15 minutes until the peaches are soft and slightly caramelized.
5. Set out warm with a dollop of Greek yogurt on top.

Nutrition Information (per serving):

Calories: 90, Total Fat: 0g, Carbohydrates: 22g, Fiber: 3g, Protein: 2g

Chia Seed Pudding with Berries

Servings: 2

Prep Time: 5 minutes

Chilling Time: 2 hours or overnight

Ingredients:

- 1/4 cup chia seeds
- 1 cup unsweetened milk or coconut milk
- 1 tablespoon honey or maple syrup
- Fresh berries for topping

Directions:

1. In a bowl, mix chia seeds, almond/coconut milk, and honey/maple syrup. Stir well.
2. Let it sit for a few minutes, then stir again to prevent clumps.
3. Lid and refrigerate for at least 2 hours or overnight, allowing it to thicken.
4. Before serving, stir the pudding and top with fresh berries.

Nutrition Information (per serving):

Calories: 150, Total Fat: 8g, Carbohydrates: 15g, Fiber: 10g, Protein: 5g

Fruit Kabobs

Serving: 2 kabobs

Prep Time: 15 minutes

Ingredients:

- Assorted pancreatitis-friendly fruits (such as strawberries, pineapple chunks, melon balls)
- Wooden skewers

Directions:

1. Wash and prepare the fruits, cutting them into bite-sized pieces.
2. Thread the fruit pieces onto the wooden skewers in an alternating pattern.
3. Serve it strainght away or refrigerate until ready to serve.

Nutrition Information:

Nutritional value varies based on fruit selection. Generally, low in fat and sodium, high in vitamins and fiber.

Chocolate Covered Strawberries

Serving: 4 strawberries

Prep Time: 20 minutes

Cook Time: 5 minutes

Ingredients:

- 8 fresh strawberries (washed and dried)
- 1/2 cup dark chocolate chips (pancreatitis-friendly)
- Optional: Chopped nuts or shredded coconut for garnish

Directions:

1. Lay a tray or plate with parchment paper.
2. Into a microwave-safe bowl, melt the dark chocolate chips in 30-second intervals, mixing between each interval until smooth.
3. Coat each strawberry into the melted chocolate, coating it halfway. Place them on the prepared tray.
4. If desired, sprinkle chopped nuts or shredded coconut on the chocolate-coated strawberries.
5. Refrigerate for 15-20 minutes until the chocolate hardens.

Nutrition Information:

Varies based on the amount of chocolate used. Dark chocolate may offer antioxidants and moderate sugar content.

Greek Yogurt Parfait

Serving: 1-2 servings

Prep Time: 10 minutes

Ingredients:

- 1 cup pancreatitis-friendly Greek yogurt
- Fresh or canned berries (such as blueberries or raspberries)
- Granola (low-fat, low-sugar variety)

Directions:

1. Take a glass or bowl, layer Greek yogurt, followed by a layer of berries, and a sprinkle of granola.
2. Repeat the layers as desired.
3. Serve immediately.

Nutrition Information:

Rich in protein, calcium, and probiotics from Greek yogurt. Nutritional content depends on the granola used.

Rice Pudding

Serving: 2 servings

Prep Time: 5 minutes

Cook Time: 30 minutes

Ingredients:

- 1/2 cup white rice
- 2 cups low-fat milk or lactose-free milk
- 2 tablespoons sugar or sweetener (if allowed)
- 1/2 teaspoon vanilla extract
- Cinnamon (optional for flavor)

Directions:

1. Rinse the rice thoroughly.

2. In a saucepan, combine rice, milk, sugar/sweetener, and vanilla extract.
3. Bring to a simmer down over medium-low heat, stirring at times.
4. Cook for 25-30 minutes or until the rice is tender and the mixture thickens.
5. Remove from heat and let it cool. Sprinkle with cinnamon if desired before serving.

Nutrition Information:

Moderate in carbohydrates and protein, low in fat.

Baked Banana Chips

Serving: 1-2 servings

Prep Time: 10 minutes

Cook Time: 2-3 hours (baking time)

Ingredients:

- 2 ripe but firm bananas
- Lemon juice (optional, to prevent browning)

Directions:

1. Set the oven to 200°F (93°C). Line a baking sheet with parchment paper.
2. Slice the bananas into thin rounds. If desired, lightly brush the slices with lemon juice to prevent browning.
3. Put the banana slices on the prepared baking sheet in a single layer.
4. Bake for 2-3 hours, flipping the slices halfway through, until they are crispy.
5. Let them cool completely before serving.

Nutrition Information:

Low in fat, a good source of potassium and fiber.

Homemade Applesauce

Servings: 2

Prep Time: 10 minutes

Cook Time: 15 minutes

Ingredients:

- 4 apples (peeled, cored, and chopped)
- 1 tablespoon lemon juice
- 1 teaspoon ground cinnamon
- 1/4 cup water

Directions:

1. Place the chopped apples, lemon juice, cinnamon, and water in a saucepan over medium heat.
2. Lid and cook for 10-15 minutes until the apples are soft, stirring occasionally.
3. Once softened, mash the apples using a fork or blend for a smoother consistency.
4. Let it cool before serving. Store leftovers in the refrigerator.

Nutrition Information (per serving):

Calories: 90, Total Fat: 0g, Cholesterol: 0mg, Sodium: 0mg, Total Carbohydrates: 24g, Dietary Fiber: 5g, Sugars: 18g, Protein: 0g

Frozen Fruit Cups

Servings: 2

Prep Time: 10 minutes

Freezing Time: 2-3 hours

Ingredients:

- 1 cup mixed fruits (such as berries, grapes, and diced apples)

- 1/2 cup unsweetened fruit juice (like apple or orange juice)

Directions:

1. Mix the fruits in a bowl and evenly distribute them into two cupcake liners or small cups.
2. Pour the fruit juice over the fruits until they're just covered.
3. Place in the freezer for 2-3 hours until completely frozen.
4. Serve as a refreshing frozen treat.

Nutrition Information (per serving):

Calories: 70, Total Fat: 0g, Cholesterol: 0mg, Sodium: 0mg, Total Carbohydrates: 18g, Dietary Fiber: 3g, Sugars: 13g, Protein: 1g

Berry Smoothie Bowl

Servings: 1

Prep Time: 5 minutes

Ingredients:

- 1 cup mixed berries (fresh or frozen)
- 1 ripe banana
- 1/2 cup plain yogurt (low-fat or non-fat)
- 2 tablespoons honey (optional for sweetness)
- Toppings: sliced almonds, shredded coconut, additional berries (optional)

Directions:

1. Blend the mixed berries, banana, yogurt, and honey (if using) until smooth.
2. Pour the smoothie into a bowl.
3. Top with sliced almonds, shredded coconut, and additional berries if desired.
4. Serve immediately.

Nutrition Information:

Calories: 300, Total Fat: 4g, Cholesterol: 5mg, Sodium: 60mg, Total Carbohydrates: 65g, Dietary Fiber: 10g, Sugars: 44g, Protein: 8g

Peach Cobbler

Servings: 2

Prep Time: 10 minutes

Cook Time: 25 minutes

Ingredients:

- 2 cups sliced peaches (fresh or canned in juice)
- 1/2 teaspoon ground cinnamon
- 1/4 teaspoon nutmeg
- 1 tablespoon honey
- 1/2 cup rolled oats
- 2 tablespoons melted butter (unsalted)

Directions:

1. Set out the oven to 350°F (175°C).
2. In a bowl, mix the peaches, cinnamon, nutmeg, and honey. Place the mixture in a baking dish.
3. In another bowl, combine the rolled oats and melted butter. Sprinkle this mixture over the peach mixture.
4. Cook it for 25 minutes or until the topping is golden brown.
5. Allow it to cool slightly before serving.

Nutrition Information (per serving):

Calories: 220, Total Fat: 9g, Cholesterol: 15mg, Sodium: 55mg, Total Carbohydrates: 36g, Dietary Fiber: 5g, Sugars: 24g, Protein: 3g

Servings: 2

Prep Time: 15 minutes

Cook Time: 10 minutes

Ingredients:

For Fruit Salsa:

- 1 cup diced mixed fruits (such as strawberries, kiwi, and pineapple)
- 1 tablespoon fresh lime juice
- 1 tablespoon honey
- 1 teaspoon fresh mint leaves (chopped)

For Cinnamon Chips:

- 2 whole wheat tortillas
- Cooking spray
- 1 tablespoon sugar
- 1/2 teaspoon ground cinnamon

Directions:

1. In a bowl, mix the diced fruits, lime juice, honey, and chopped mint leaves. Set aside.
2. Set out the oven to 350°F (175°C).
3. Cut each tortilla into wedges. Put on a baking sheet, spray with cooking spray, and sprinkle with sugar and cinnamon.
4. Bake for 8-10 minutes or until the tortilla chips are crispy.
5. Serve the fruit salsa with the cinnamon chips for dipping.

Nutrition Information (per serving):

Calories: 180, Total Fat: 3g, Cholesterol: 0mg, Sodium: 150mg, Total Carbohydrates: 38g, Dietary Fiber: 4g, Sugars: 18g, Protein: 3g

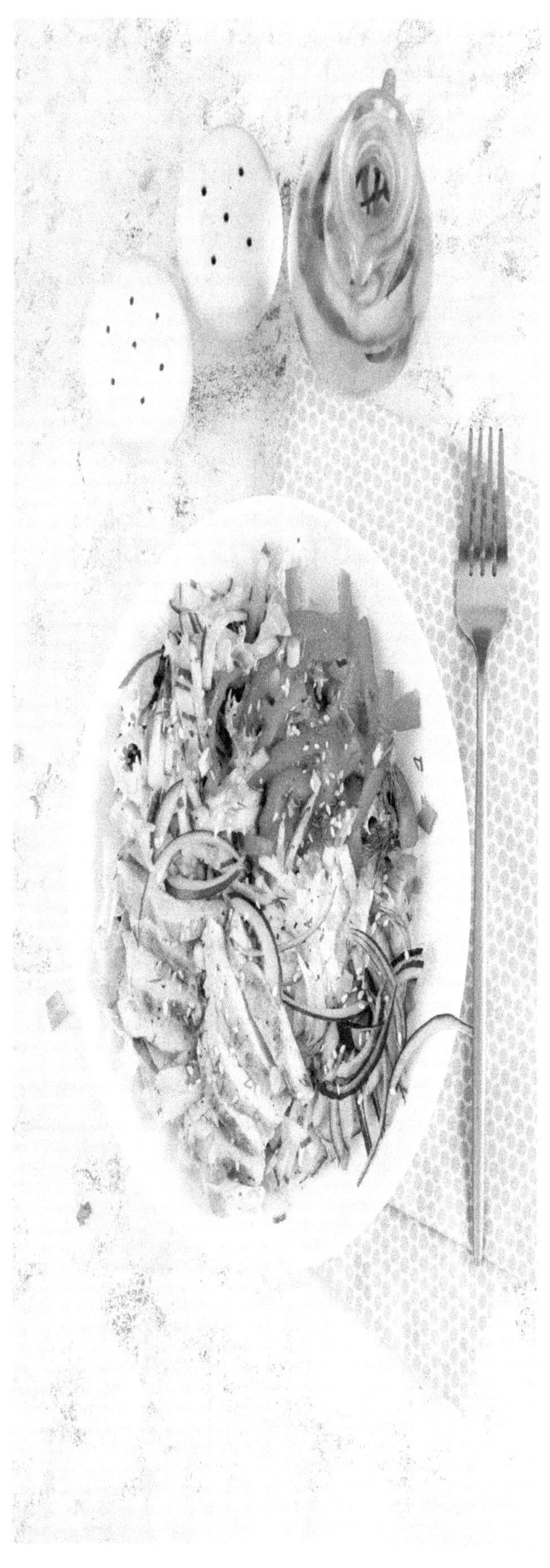

The Pancreatitis Diet stands out from other dietary plans due to its specific focus on alleviating symptoms and promoting healing in the pancreas—a vital organ responsible for generating digestive enzymes and insulin. Pancreatitis occurs when the pancreas turns into inflamed, leading to digestive complications and potential long-term health issues.

Here's how the Pancreatitis Diet differs from other diets:

★ Low Fat Emphasis:

Unlike many popular diets, the Pancreatitis Diet typically involves a strict restriction of fat intake. Fat can trigger the release of digestive enzymes, putting strain on the inflamed pancreas. This diet prioritizes low-fat foods to reduce this burden and ease pancreatic inflammation.

★ Moderation in Protein Intake:

While protein is essential, excessive consumption can also stress the pancreas. The diet recommends moderate protein intake, usually from lean sources like chicken, fish, tofu, and legumes, to aid in tissue repair without overworking the pancreas.

★ Avoidance of Trigger Foods:

Certain foods can exacerbate symptoms of pancreatitis. These include fatty and fried foods, high-fat dairy, red meat, processed foods, and those high in refined sugars. The diet plan focuses on eliminating or minimizing these trigger foods to prevent flare-ups.

★ Emphasis on Fresh, Whole Foods:

A significant aspect of the Pancreatitis Diet involves incorporating fresh fruits, vegetables, whole grains, and healthy fats (in limited quantities) like avocados and nuts. These foods provide vital nutrients and antioxidants that aid in reducing inflammation and promoting healing.

★ Hydration and Alcohol Avoidance:

Staying well-hydrated is crucial for pancreatic health. The diet encourages ample water intake while strictly avoiding alcohol, which can further inflame the pancreas and hinder recovery.

★ Small, Frequent Meals:

Instead of three large meals, the diet recommends consuming smaller, more frequent meals throughout the day. This eases the digestive workload on the pancreas and helps manage blood sugar level.

★ Medical Supervision and Individualization:

It's important to note that the Pancreatitis Diet may vary among individuals based on the severity of the condition, personal health history, and other factors. Hence, it's crucial to seek guidance from a healthcare professional or a registered nutritionist who specializes in pancreatitis to create a tailored diet plan.

By focusing on low-fat, easily digestible foods, limiting triggers, and emphasizing hydration and nutrient-rich options, the Pancreatitis Diet aims to support the healing process, manage symptoms, and prevent complications associated with pancreatic inflammation.

When dealing with pancreatitis, it's crucial to approach diet and exercises with caution, as the condition involves inflammation of the pancreas.

Here are five steps for a pancreatitis diet and exercises:

Consultation with a Healthcare Professional

Before starting any diet or exercise regimen for pancreatitis, it's essential to consult with a healthcare professional. They can supply personalized guidance based on the severity and type of pancreatitis you have. A registered dietitian or nutritionist specializing in pancreatic health can create a tailored plan.

Pancreatitis Diet Guidelines

★ **Low-Fat Diet:**

A primary focus of the pancreatitis diet is reducing fat intake. High-fat foods can trigger pancreas inflammation. Choose lean proteins like chicken, turkey, fish, and legumes. Limit saturated fats form in red meat and full-fat dairy.

★ **Small, Frequent Meals:**

Eating smaller, more recurrent meals throughout the day instead of three large meals can ease digestion and reduce stress on the pancreas.

★ **Emphasize Fruits and Vegetables:**

These are rich in vitamins, minerals, and antioxidants. Opt for a variety of rich fruits and vegetables to obtain essential nutrients.

★ **Avoid Alcohol and Caffeine:**

Both can irritate the pancreas, worsening inflammation. It's crucial to eliminate or significantly reduce alcohol and caffeine intake.

Hydration and Lifestyle Changes

★ **Stay Hydrated:**

Proper hydration is crucial for pancreatic health. Aim to drink sufficient amount of water throughout the day, but avoid sugary beverages.

★ **Avoid Smoking:**

Smoking can aggravate pancreatitis. If you smoke, quitting is highly recommended to reduce inflammation and improve overall health.

★ **Manage Stress:**

Stress can worsen symptoms. Engage in stress-reducing movements like meditation, yoga, or deep breathing exercises.

Safe Exercises for Pancreatitis

★ **Low-Impact Activities:**

Walking, swimming, cycling, and gentle yoga are excellent low-impact exercises suitable for individuals with pancreatitis. These activities promote circulation and overall well-being without putting excessive strain on the body.

★ **Gradual Progression:**

Start slowly and steadily increase the intensity and duration of exercise. Listen to your body and prevent movements that cause discomfort or pain in the abdominal area.

Regular Monitoring and Adaptation

* **Regular Check-ups:**

Schedule regular follow-ups with your healthcare provider to monitor your condition and make necessary adjustments to your diet and exercise routine.

* **Adapt as Needed:**

If you experience any changes in symptoms or have concerns about your diet or exercise plan, discuss them with your healthcare team. They can provide guidance on modifications that may be necessary.

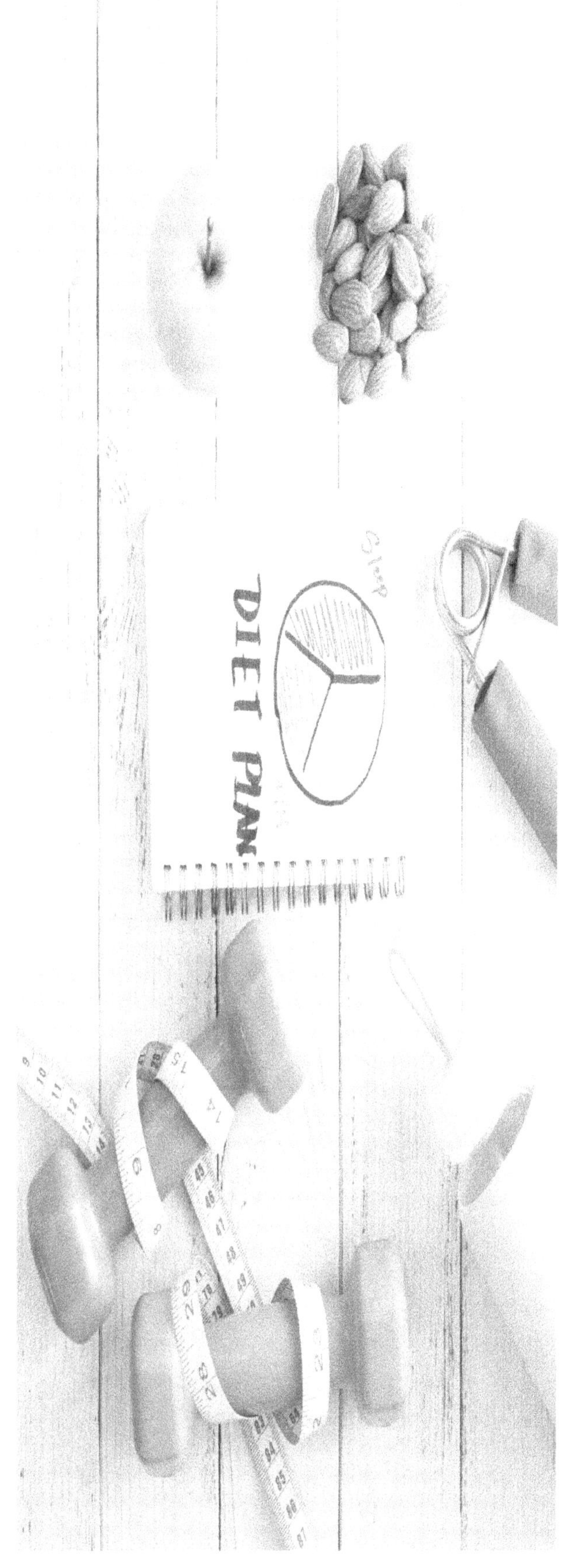

21 Days Meal Plan

Week 1

Day	Breakfast	Lunch	Snack	Dinner
Monday	Oatmeal with Blueberries	Quinoa and Black Bean Salad	Fruit Salad	Baked Cod with Herbs
Tuesday	Banana Walnut Pancakes	Miso Soup with Tofu and Vegetables	Vegetable Sticks with Hummus	Spinach and Feta Stuffed Mushrooms
Wednesday	Egg White Veggie Omelette	Tuna Salad Lettuce Wraps	Greek Yogurt with Berries	Cucumber Dill Salad
Thursday	Fruit Salad	Brown Rice Stir-Fry	Rice Cakes with Almond Butter	Cauliflower Mash
Friday	Greek Yogurt Parfait	Vegetable Lentil Soup	Baked Apple Chips	Sweet Potato Rounds
Saturday	Whole Wheat Toast with Almond Butter	Hummus and Veggie Sandwich	Cottage Cheese with Pineapple	Greek Yogurt Dip with Veggies
Sunday	Quinoa Breakfast Bowl	Caprese Salad	Whole Grain Crackers with Avocado	Greek Orzo Salad

Week 2

Day	Breakfast	Lunch	Snack	Dinner
Monday	Smoothie	Grilled Vegetable Salad	Fruit Smoothie	Baked Lemon Herb Chicken
Tuesday	Cottage Cheese with Pineapple	Turkey and Veggie Wrap	Vegetable Chips	Vegetable Stir-Fry with Tofu
Wednesday	Muesli with Low-Fat Milk	Sweet Potato and Chickpea Salad	Chia Seed Pudding	Salmon and Asparagus Foil Packets
Thursday	Veggie Breakfast Burrito	Zucchini Noodles with Marinara Sauce	Hummus Cucumber Bites	Mushroom and Spinach Pasta
Friday	Baked Apple with Cinnamon	Broccoli and Cauliflower Soup	Frozen Grapes	Roasted Vegetable and Quinoa Bowl
Saturday	Avocado Toast	Egg Salad Lettuce Wraps	Baked Tortilla Chips with Salsa	Black Bean and Corn Tacos
Sunday	Rice Cake with Hummus	Vegetable Quiche	Apple Slices with Almond Butter	Eggplant Parmesan

Day	Breakfast	Lunch	Snack	Dinner
Monday	Steamed Vegetables with Tofu	Brown Rice and Bean Burrito Bowl	Low-Fat Yogurt Parfait	Veggie and Bean Chili
Tuesday	Chia Seed Pudding	Greek Salad with Grilled Chicken	Celery and Peanut Butter	Grilled Shrimp Skewers
Wednesday	Whole Grain Waffles with Berries	Cauliflower Rice Stir-Fry	Roasted Chickpeas	Vegetable Curry
Thursday	Brown Rice Porridge	Salmon Salad	Fruit Skewers	Lentil and Vegetable Stew
Friday	Spinach and Feta Frittata	Tofu Lettuce Wraps	Homemade Applesauce	Cauliflower Steaks
Saturday	Low-Fat Bran Muffins	Vegetable Pasta Primavera	Frozen Fruit Cups	Quinoa Stuffed Bell Peppers
Sunday	Ginger Carrot Soup	Baked Lemon Herb Chicken Breast	Berry Smoothie Bowl	Turkey Meatballs with Marinara

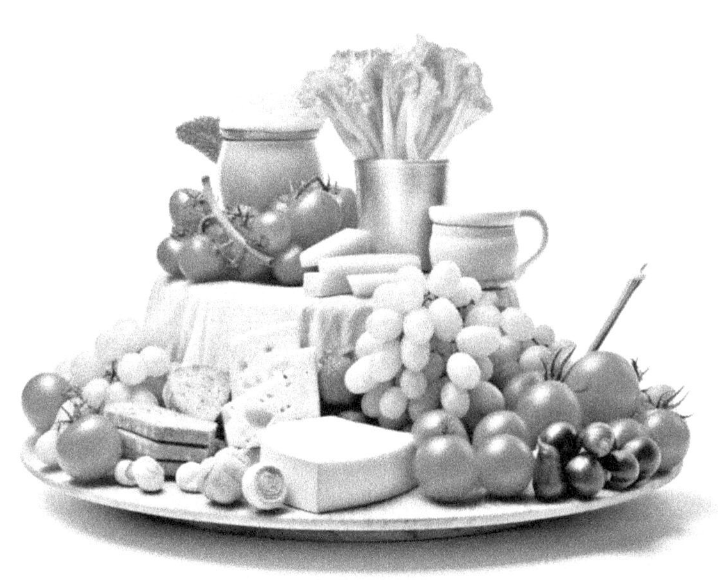

Individuals navigating through pancreatitis, offering a collection of nutritious, delicious recipes tailored to support pancreatic health. Pancreatitis is a complex condition that requires careful attention to dietary choices to manage symptoms and promote healing.

Throughout this cookbook, we've explored the significance of a well-thought-out diet in managing pancreatitis. By focusing on nutrient-dense, easily digestible foods, individuals can potentially alleviate discomfort, reduce inflammation, and support the pancreas in its healing process.

The recipes included in this book have been meticulously crafted to adhere to the dietary guidelines recommended for pancreatitis management. Emphasizing low-fat, low-spice, and easily digestible ingredients, these recipes aim to offer variety without compromising on flavor or nutritional value.

Moreover, we've highlighted the importance of consulting with healthcare professionals or registered dietitians before making significant dietary changes, especially for individuals dealing with pancreatitis. Every individual's situation is unique, and personalized guidance ensures that dietary adjustments align with specific health needs and considerations.

By incorporating a diverse compass of nutrient-rich foods, such as lean proteins, whole grains, fruits, vegetables, and healthy fats in appropriate portions, individuals can create meals that not only support pancreatitis management but also contribute to overall well-being.

Furthermore, the emphasis on hydration cannot be overstated. Adequate water intake plays a vital role in maintaining optimal health and aiding digestion, factors crucial in managing pancreatitis symptoms.

In essence, this cookbook is intended as a tool to empower individuals with pancreatitis to take charge of their dietary habits, encouraging a balanced approach that supports healing, reduces discomfort, and enhances quality of life. While dietary adjustments are an integral part of managing pancreatitis, it's essential to complement these changes with medical guidance, a healthy lifestyle, and ongoing self-care practices.

May this cookbook serve as a valuable resource on the journey toward better health and well-being for those navigating the challenges of pancreatitis. Remember, making informed, mindful food choices can significantly impact one's health and vitality, fostering a path toward a brighter, healthier future.